ADVERSE REACTIONS TO DRUGS

ADVERSE REACTIONS TO DRUGS

SECOND EDITION

by

O. L. WADE, M.A.(Cantab.), M.D., F.R.C.P.(Lond.), Hon.F.R.C.P.I.
Professor of Therapeutics and Clinical Pharmacology, University of Birmingham
Member of the Medicine Commission and previously a member of the Committee on Safety of Drugs

and

LINDA BEELEY, M.A.(Oxon.), M.R.C.P.
Lecturer in Therapeutics and Clinical Pharmacology, University of Birmingham

LONDON
WILLIAM HEINEMANN MEDICAL BOOKS LTD

First published 1970
Reprinted 1973
Second Edition 1976

ISBN 0 433 34551 9

Printed and bound in Great Britain by R. J. Acford Ltd., Industrial Estate,
Chichester, Sussex

CONTENTS

PREFACE TO THE SECOND EDITION

The first edition of this book was published in 1970. In mid 1973 a new edition was needed and I decided to revise the book. It soon became clear however that so much had happened in the field of adverse reactions to drugs that revision was impractical: the book needed rewriting. The task of rewriting has given me the opportunity not only of recasting the subject matter and altering the emphasis of the book but also of inviting Dr. Linda Beeley to join me as a co-author. She became a member of the staff of the Department of Therapeutics of Birmingham University shortly after I had moved here from Queen's University of Belfast in 1971 and it is a pleasure for me to acknowledge the contribution she has made to the book from her extensive knowledge of adverse reactions to drugs.

The only feature of the book which we have not changed is its plan. The book starts with a short account of adverse reactions to drugs and the problems they present to doctors and dentists, to the drug industry and to governmental agencies. The second part of the book consists of appendices containing compilations of adverse reactions to drugs. These are arranged to be convenient for easy reference. The lists are not completely comprehensive, for otherwise this small paperback pygmy would become a giant and would lose much of its value to the reader. The first part of the book is meant to stimulate interest in adverse reactions to drugs: the second part, the appendices, is meant to be of help to doctors in their daily work. It is not meant to be a textbook or a reference book, but we give a short bibliography so that the reader may seek further and more detailed information if he wishes.

Most serious adverse reactions to drugs are uncommon and no single doctor is likely to have extensive experience of them. For this reason it is extremely important that we should all report any serious or unexpected adverse reactions to drugs, especially new drugs, to the Committee on Safety of Medicines. This is the main way in which the medical community can be made aware of previously unsuspected adverse reactions and by which our knowledge of the frequency and seriousness of known reactions can be increased. Had it not been for reports from doctors it would never have been possible to identify that the oestrogen content of oral contraceptives was the important factor in determining the incidence of thromboembolic complications, the hazards of bronchodilator aerosols would not have been suspected and the unacceptable incidence of jaundice caused by certain anti-inflammatory analgesic drugs might not have been detected. All of us dislike the chore of filling in forms but these reports to the Committee on Safety of Medicines are needed if patients are to be protected and colleagues are to be helped.

ACKNOWLEDGMENTS

We are indebted to many colleagues in both Belfast and Birmingham for comment and criticism but most especially to Mervyn Mitchard and Martin Kendall who not only read early drafts of the revision of the book but gave us much encouragement and support in our task.

We are grateful to Miss Robin Wade who designed the book cover and deeply indebted to Mr. R. S. Emery of William Heinemann Medical Books Ltd., for his courtesy, kindness and patience in preparing our typescript for publication.

CHAPTER I

THE DAWN OF CONCERN

Doctors have always known that the treatment or remedies they give their patients may do harm instead of good. Indeed in ancient Mesopotamia this was recognised in the legal system and the Code of Hammurabi enforced grim punishments on the doctor if perchance the harm was due to his incompetence.

Fifteen hundred years later Hippocrates was also aware that treatment might do harm. He enjoined the physician to study man, to treat suffering with compassion and to accept the axiom of *non nocere* as a basis for his therapy. The great humane ideals of the Hippocratic tradition did not persist. The slanders and controversies that troubled medieval medicine in Europe make fascinating reading. A persistent theme of most physicians is that their own remedies are valuable but those of their colleagues harmful. Self criticism did not come easily and there is seldom any suggestion that their own remedies might do harm.

George Washington the first President of the United States fell ill in the last year of the eighteenth century. He had been riding around his estate on the banks of the Potomac River in a rainstorm and returned to sit down to lunch, an extensive meal that lasted from 1 to 5 p.m., drenching wet. That evening he had a sore throat, which from reading the accounts might have been streptococcal or diphtheritic. His physicians set to energetically. He was given gargles of molasses vinegar and butter and of vinegar and sage tea, cantharides was applied to his neck to produce blisters and he was bled heavily four times "his strength meanwhile rapidly sinking". If he had lived it would seem to us now that this would have been despite the treatment: as it was he died on 14th December 1799. His doctors were not fools. They were intelligent men trying hard to do their best for a popular and much loved leader. The blisters, the purges and the extensive bleeding were all done to remove the evil humours which since Galen's time were thought to be the cause of disease.

Thirty years later Charles Louis at the Charité Hospital, Paris, was one of the first physicians to question these heroic measures and carry out scientific measurements of their value. He examined the effects of bleeding in patients with pneumonia. Louis concluded that the longer bleeding was delayed the better the outcome for the patient and he suggested the outcome might be better still if no blood at all was let. His anguish at finding that a widely accepted and valued therapeutic procedure might do harm and not good to his patients is apparent in the introduction of the short paper in which he published his results (Louis, 1828).

> "Le résultat de mes recherches sur les effets de la saignée dans les inflammations est si peu d'accord avec l'opinion commune, que ce n'est pas sans une sorte d'hésitation que je me suis décidé a les exposer. Après avoir analysé une première fois les faits qui y sont relatifs, j'ai cru m'etre trompé, et j'ai recommencé mon travail; mais les résultats de cette nouvelle analyse restant toujours les mêmes . . ."

Despite these observations, Louis found to his dismay that blood letting was so firmly established that to fail to let blood in a serious illness was regarded as professional negligence. His dilemma is not unique. There have been many instances in modern times when therapy has been demonstrated to be of no use or to be hazardous, but this does not mean that it ceases to be used. Long term anticoagulants are still used in coronary disease, antibiotics are still widely prescribed for minor upper respiratory tract virus infections, and chloramphenicol continues to be used for minor infections long after the hazards of aplastic anaemia have been recognised.

Chloroform was first used as an anaesthetic by Flourens in 1847 in animals and in the same year James Simpson of

Edinburgh first used it in humans. It was a much more pleasant anaesthetic to administer than ether and in those days of open fires and oil lights much safer. But as its use increased it was found that occasionally patients died unexpectedly and suddenly during the induction of anaesthesia. This was often tragic if a young fit person undergoing a minor surgical procedure died and there was considerable concern about it. In 1877 the British Medical Association appointed a committee to investigate these deaths. Investigations were carried out in animals and reports of fatal accidents in patients were analysed. The committee published three interim reports and its final report, published in 1880, was signed by John G. McKendrick, Professor of Physiology, Joseph Coates, Pathologist and David Newman, Pathological Chemist, all of Glasgow. They found that chloroform was hazardous not only because in large doses it caused respiratory depression but because it also had deleterious effects on the heart and even in small doses, at the beginning of induction, it might cause cardiac arrest. This investigation is the first major collaborative investigation of the adverse reactions of a drug ever carried out. It is still well worth while reading the well documented report: no other investigation of adverse reactions of drugs of comparable scientific calibre was to be carried out for another forty years.

The unexpected deaths from chloroform were few and far between and many doctors who used chloroform had never seen one of these unfortunate accidents, so that when the BMA report was published, there were many who dissented from its findings. Amongst these was Surgeon Major E. Lawrie, Residency Surgeon at Hyderabad in India. Lawrie had been a student at Edinburgh and had studied under James Simpson who introduced chloroform. He appointed the Hyderabad Chloroform Commission with himself as President. The four members of the Commission carried out a number of experiments on dogs and in 1889 reported that "chloroform may be given to dogs by inhalation with perfect safety and without any fear of accidental death if only the respiration and nothing but the respiration is carefully attended to throughout". This report was short, was presented without any supporting data and had a sceptical and scathing reception from the *Lancet* (Annotation, 1889; Leader, 1889). Correspondence between Lawrie and the Editor of the *Lancet* followed and reading the letters in the old journals one is surprised that the yellowed pages are not charred, so heated and vitriolic is the language.

The controversy led to the appointment of the Second Hyderabad Chloroform Commission of which Lawrie was the President and Dr. Brunton, F.R.S., appointed as a member on behalf of the *Lancet*. Extensive investigations were carried out in dogs which convincingly vindicated Lawrie for there was no evidence that chloroform specifically affected the heart. A report was published (Lawrie, Brunton, Bomford and Hakim, 1890) which claimed, in the words of a contemporary Anglo-Indian "that chloroform was as safe as whisky and water". But this report carried little weight for by this time the clinical evidence that chloroform could in humans cause sudden and unexpected cardiac arrest was unequivocal. In retrospect this episode is one of the first demonstrations that pharmacological studies done in animals are not necessarily applicable in man. It is now recognised that chloroform sensitises the myocardium to catecholamines which may induce a variety of cardiac arrythmias including fatal ventricular fibrillation, and that this is a hazard during the induction of anaesthesia in a nervous patient who has had inadequate premedication.

During the first world war there was an outbreak of jaundice at Cherry Hinton Military Hospital near Cambridge. The hospital was a centre for the treatment of venereal disease and neoarsphenamine benzoate, salvarsan, which was used to treat syphilis was suspected of causing hepatic damage. A number of patients died of acute yellow atrophy and official concern was so great that the Medical Research Committee, later to become the Medical Research Council was asked to investigate the catastrophe. A "Special committee on the manufacture, biological testing and clinical administration of salvarsan and its substitutes" was appointed with Sir Humphrey Rolleston as Chairman. Although the Committee reported (Medical Research Council, 1922) that the most probable cause of the outbreak was the hepatic toxicity of the organo-arsenical compounds, one of its members, Stuart McDonald, Professor of Pathology at Newcastle, suspected that there was an additional factor which had caused the epidemic-like outbreak of jaundice at Cherry Hinton (McDonald, 1918) and he thought this was a microbial infection. In retrospect McDonald was probably right and it is likely the soldiers suffered syringe borne serum hepatitis, a disease which was not to be identified until a second World War was upon us. McDonald's suspicions might well have been confirmed if the Committee had taken closer note of another outbreak of illness which it was asked to investigate at Portobello Hospital, Dublin. Portobello was another venereal disease centre at which intensive intravenous neoarsphenamine therapy had replaced the more usual long continued intermittent intramuscular injections of the drug. Eight soldiers given this treatment died of malaria although only one of them had ever served in a tropical country. Professor O'Sullivan, the Professor of Pathology at Trinity College, found their organs full of malarial parasites and suggested that the infection had been conveyed from one or more persons infected with malaria to the others by the apparatus of administering the arsphenamine infusion, the blood of the carrier regurgitating into the last segments of the tubing of the infusion apparatus, remaining in the crevices there and being washed into the veins of the next patient. The transferance of the virus of serum hepatitis by syringe is not very different and the Committee came very near to identifying the hazard of transmitting infective jaundice from patient to patient.

Cincophen is an analgesic drug which was introduced to medical practice in 1908 and was widely used to relieve the pain of rheumatoid arthritis and gout. It was not until 1923, however, that a London physician (Worster-Drought, 1923) first described severe jaundice in a patient who had taken a total of 16G of cincophen in 71 days. After his report others followed (Rake, 1927; Short & Bauer, 1933) but cincophen remained a drug that could be purchased by the public without prescription and at an inquest in Birmingham in 1934 several doctors denied that they had ever heard of cincophen causing jaundice, although this denial did appear to surprise the coroner. Again and again it is surprising how long it is after the marketing of a drug before its adverse reactions are recognised, and how unevenly information about adverse reaction spreads amongst doctors, so that many years later after an adverse reaction has been widely recognised and discussed, there will still be some who have not heard of it.

There was a long interval between the introduction of amidopyrine as an analgesic in 1889 and recognition that it caused agranulocytosis. It was not until 1933 that Madison and Squier suggested amidopyrine and other drugs containing a benzene ring might cause agranulocytosis. The confirmation came from an astute piece of epidemiological observation. Kracke and Parker (1934) observed that agranulocytosis was surprisingly common amongst nurses and doctors. It was then easily ascertained that a high proportion of those who had developed agranulocytosis were in the habit of resorting to analgesic preparations containing amidopyrine. Over the counter sales of amidopyrine were prohibited in Britain in 1936 and in the U.S.A. in 1938. The drug is however still widely available without a doctor's prescription in other European countries and most of the patients developing agranulocytosis due to amidopyrine reported to the Committee on Safety of Medicines have been unsuspecting tourists who have purchased the drug when on holiday. In France and many other countries amidopyrine is still considered a useful remedy and is widely used: why the natives of these countries should be able to take the drug with impunity is one of the minor mysteries of adverse reactions to drugs. Similarly, chloramphenicol which is widely used in West Germany does not seem to be as serious a cause of aplastic anaemia there as it is in Britain and the U.S.A.

Adverse reactions to vaccines and antisera have always attracted considerable public attention and anxiety. The anxiety has often been heightened by the emotional accusations of anti-vaccinationists and anti-vivisectionists. One of the first recorded large scale catastrophes occurred in August 1883 when 1,350 men working in a shipyard at Bremen were vaccinated against smallpox with glycerinated human lymph and 191 subsequently suffered jaundice.

There was a wide public concern in 1928 when a bottle of diphtheria toxin-antitoxin mixture was contaminated with staphylococcus pyogenes and 12 out of 21 children inoculated from it died in Bundaberg, Queensland. And in 1930 a tragic accident at Lubeck in Germany caused a considerable setback to B.C.G. immunisation campaigns throughout the world. By error a culture of virulent human tubercle bacilli was fed to 250 infants. Over a quarter of them died.

But the most notorious of all vaccine catastrophes was the Cutter incident. It occurred in the U.S.A. at a time when poliomyelitis was the subject of public fear and anxiety. Over a 10-day period in mid-April, 1955, about 400,000 persons, mostly schoolchildren, had been inoculated, as part of a nationwide campaign against poliomyelitis, with vaccine made by the Cutter Laboratories, Berkeley, California. On April 25th an infant was admitted to a Chicago hospital with paralytic poliomyelitis. This child had been inoculated with Cutter vaccine on April 16th. The next day poliomyelitis was reported in five more children who had received Cutter vaccine and in the next 2 months 260 cases were reported, 94 in vaccinees, 126 in the family contacts of the vaccinees and 40 among contacts in the community. Investigation showed that two batches of the formaldehyde inactivated Salk type Cutter vaccine contained living poliomyelitis virus. Although it was found that there had been no negligence the Company were liable under the American laws of warranty and paid out $3 million in compensation.

Awareness of adverse reactions to drugs forced itself upon doctors when the sulphonamides were introduced. In 1935 Domagh described the effectiveness of the dye *prontosil rubra* in the treatment of experimental streptococcal infections. This dye had been first synthesised by Gelmo in 1908. Its value in human puerpural fever was convincingly demonstrated by Colebrook and Kenny (1936) and subsequently a number of related sulphonamides were extensively used. The sulphonamides caused many adverse reactions including renal damage, haemolysis, rashes and the unpleasant Stevens Johnson Syndrome. But such were the dramatic benefits of the sulpha drugs in the days before antibiotics that these toxic effects although recognised were accepted. It was much the same when penicillin, streptomycin and cortisone were later introduced. The benefits derived from these drugs were obvious. Adverse reactions even though sometimes fatal or so severe that therapy had to be withdrawn, were acceptable and this state of affairs continued without question until 1961.

At a congress of gynaecologists at Kiel on 19th and 20th October 1961, von Massenbach from Lubeck, Lenz from Hamburg and Wiedemann from Kiel drew attention to the large number of children born in the previous ten months with hypoplastic or aplastic limb deformities. Such deformaties had previously been rare. Dr. Wiedemann expressed anxiety that some exogenous cause might have begun to operate and thought that it might be one of the many new drugs which were at the time being marketed. It was Dr. Lenz at a paediatric meeting in Dusseldorf on 19th November 1961, who first suggested that Contergan, a proprietary brand of thalidomide, might be the responsible agent. There were immediate consultations between Dr. Lenz, Dr. Koll, Chairman of the Drug Commission of the German Medical Association, officers of the Ministry of the Interior, North Rhineland and Westphalia and the Chief of Clinical research of Chemie Grünenthal who manufactured and marketed thalidomide. The firm withdrew thalidomide from the market on 25th November 1961.

Thalidomide was first marketed as *Contergan,* a safe non-barbiturate hypnotic in West Germany in 1956 and in Britain in 1958 as *Distaval.* Within a short time it was marketed throughout Western Europe under a number of proprietary names and it was included with analgesics in many compound tablets for the treatment of pain, cough and insomnia. Many of these preparations which were skilfully promoted, became widely prescribed by doctors and in West Germany many were extensively purchased by members of the public. The profusion of proprietary names was to make retrospective enquiries about the drugs women had used in pregnancy difficult, but investigations soon confirmed Dr. Lenz's suspicions. In a survey in West Germany of 10 large obstetric units, it was found that in the 10 years up to 1959 no children with phocomelia or micromelia were born; in 1959 there were 10, in 1960, 26 and in 1961, 477. And in another study of 46 mothers delivered of deformed babies, 41 were found to have certainly taken thalidomide during their early pregnancy while in a control series of 300 mothers delivered of normal babies, none had taken thalidomide. Experiments with animals confirmed that thalidomide was teratogenic and if given in early pregnancy might cause limb abnormalities of the fetus (Mellin and Katzenstein, 1962).

It is now estimated that 6,000 deformed babies were born in West Germany as a result of the use of thalidomide. In Great Britain there were at least 500 live births of deformed infants. Many of these children are terribly disabled. They remain a grim reminder of a tragedy which shocked the world.

The most important result of this catastrophe was that it focussed attention on adverse reactions to drugs and in many countries governments established drug regulatory bodies to ensure that adequate and appropriate tests were done before new drugs or new pharmaceutical preparations were marketed. The dawn of concern about adverse reactions had broken; its light has increased in the intervening years but even now it does not shine in every corner.

CHAPTER II

ADVERSE REACTIONS

Many attempts have been made to define an adverse reaction to a drug. The definition used by the World Health Organisation (WHO, 1969) is that an adverse reaction is "one which is noxious, unintended and occurs at doses normally used in man for prophylaxis, diagnosis and therapy". This definition was drawn up specifically for the purpose of monitoring the adverse reactions to drugs in general clinical use, the main purpose of which is to identify unforeseen adverse reactions after a drug has been marketed. It, therefore, excludes the effects of overdose—intentional or accidental. If adhered to strictly it might also be considered to exclude the known pharmacological actions of a drug even when these are unwanted, but it is usual to include these side effects in a consideration of adverse reactions. "All systems of classifications tend in some measure to distort reality; but it is impossible to think clearly about reality unless we make some classificatory system." (Huxley, 1937.)

The following classification (Table 2.1) divides adverse

TABLE 2.1

CLASSIFICATION OF ADVERSE REACTIONS

Adverse Reactions which are Dose Related	
	Excessive Therapeutic Effect
	Side Effects — Pharmacological
	— Toxic
	Secondary Effects
Adverse Reactions which are not Dose Related	
	Idiosyncrasy
	Drug Allergy
	Unknown Mechanism
Long term Effects	
Teratogenic Effects	See chapter V page 66 *et seq.*

reactions into four main groups. Reactions in the first group are dose related and may occur in any patient who receives a drug. Their occurrence is relatively easy to predict. They constitute the vast majority of all unwanted effects of drugs, but are often more a nuisance than dangerous or serious.

Reactions in the second group are not dose related, occur in only a few individuals and are probably due to some underlying abnormality of the individual. Some are known to have an allergic basis and others are due to a well defined genetically determined abnormality, but for many the mechanism is unknown. They are much less common than the reactions in group one, and their occurrence is difficult to predict.

Dose Related Adverse Reactions to Drugs

Excessive therapeutic effect

Sometimes an adverse reaction is produced simply by an exaggeration of the normal therapeutic effect. This is most likely to occur when precise dosage is important, as is the case with the oral anticoagulants; too small a dose produces inadequate prolongation of the prothrombin time; too much may produce haemorrhage. In the treatment of diabetes insulin and the oral hypoglycaemics produce hypoglycaemia with doses not greatly above those required for adequate control of the blood sugar.

Side effects

Most drugs lack specificity. They produce a wide variety of effects within the body, acting at different receptors or on different systems. Thus the desired therapeutic effect is frequently accompanied by side effects.

Pharmacological side effects. These result from the normal pharmacological actions of a drug. They may be an extension of the main therapeutic action as are the dry mouth and blurred vision which occur when propantheline is used in the treatment of peptic ulcer; or they may be due to a pharmacological effect other than that for which the drug is being used as when a dry mouth or blurred vision are produced by a tricyclic antidepressant or chlorpromazine, or when nausea occurs with digoxin.

In a different clinical situation a side effect may become a therapeutic effect. Isoprenaline when used as a bronchodilator produces unwanted cardiac stimulation with tachycardia and the risk of arrhythmias, but in the treatment of heart block this effect is used therapeutically to increase the heart rate. When codeine is used as an analgesic, constipation is an inconvenient side effect; in the treatment of diarrhoea, however, this effect is used therapeutically.

For many drugs the dose which produces side effects is greater than the average therapeutic dose. Thus the extrapyramidal effects of chlorpromazine are usually only seen when high doses are used in the treatment of schizophrenia. In developing new drugs, or new derivatives of old drugs, attempts are made to increase specificity. Salbutamol, one of the newer bronchodilators, stimulates bronchial β adrenergic receptors at doses which have little effect on the adrenergic receptors of the heart. Prednisone is a more useful steroid than cortisone because for the same anti-inflammatory effect it produces less salt retention.

Toxic side effects. Most drugs have toxic effects if given in large enough doses. The difference between the dose required to produce a therapeutic effect and the dose which produces toxic effects is the therapeutic ratio. Drugs in which these doses are widely different have a high therapeutic ratio and rarely produce toxicity when used in therapeutic doses. For others the ratio is small and toxicity difficult to avoid, as is the case with the aminoglycoside antibiotics such as streptomycin and kanamycin which produces vestibular damage and deafness at doses very little greater than those required therapeutically. With some drugs toxicity is unavoidable; the cytotoxic drugs used in the treatment of malignant disease damage all rapidly dividing cells and depression of the bone marrow is inevitable if there is to be effective reduction in the growth of the malignant cells.

Secondary effects

These are the indirect consequences of the administration of a drug. Broad-spectrum antibiotics suppress the normal bacterial flora and encourage superinfection with resistant organisms. The lungs and bowel are most commonly involved. Thus superinfection of the bowel with candida is common during treatment with tetracyclines, and prolonged antibiotic therapy in chronic lung disease is responsible for the infections due to staphylococci and pseudomonas which occur in these patients.

Corticosteroids and immunosuppressants interfere with defence mechanisms and predispose to infection. Latent tuberculosis may become active and opportunistic infections may occur with organisms not normally pathogenic. Infections due to viruses such as cytomegalovirus, and fungi such as candida, aspergillus and cryptococcus are an important cause of death in patients requiring long term immunosuppressants after renal transplantation. A higher incidence of lymphoreticular and other tumours has also been noted in these patients, and seems to be associated particularly with the use of azathioprine.

Adverse Reactions which are not Dose Related

Idiosyncrasy

This is a term used to describe unusual reactions to drugs which occur in a few individuals. Idiosyncrasy is probably always due to some constitutional abnormality which is genetically determined but the precise mechanism of many idiosyncratic responses is unknown. Table 2.2 lists idiosyncratic reactions which are known to have a genetic basis.

Glucose-6-phosphate dehydrogenase deficiency is one of the commonest inherited enzyme defects in man, especially in American and African negroes and in some Mediterranean races. G-6-PD plays a part in the formation of reduced glutathione which is required for red cell stability and in people with G-6-PD deficiency haemolysis can be precipitated by many drugs and chemicals. In the African type of deficiency there is sufficient G-6-PD activity to prevent haemolysis of young red cells, but this activity decreases with ageing of the cells. Thus when the drug is first given haemolysis occurs but is self-limiting. As soon as the older cells have been destroyed haemolysis decreases

TABLE 2.2

IDIOSYNCRATIC DRUG REACTIONS WITH A WELL-DEFINED GENETIC BASIS

Pharmacogenetic Trait	*Adverse Effect*	*Drugs*
G-6-PD deficiency	Haemolysis	Primaquine Sulphonamides Dapsone Nitrofurantoin Aspirin Phenacetin
Methaemoglobin reductase deficiency	Methaemoglobin-aemia	Sulphonamides Phenacetin Dapsone Nitrofurantoin Primaquine Local anaesthetics— Procaine Prilocaine Nitrates, Nitrites, Chlorates
Intraocular pressure response to steroids	Glaucoma	Corticosteroids—usually topical application
Malignant hyperpyrexia	Hyperpyrexia and muscle rigidity	Suxamethonium Halothane Methoxyflurane

even if the offending drug continues to be administered. In the Mediterranean type the deficiency affects even the young cells and haemolysis tends to be more severe and prolonged. The presence of G-6-PD deficiency is thought to confer on the individual a resistance to faliciparum malaria, and the frequency of the disorder in parts of the world where malaria is endemic may be the result of natural selection of a population resistant to malaria.

With normal therapeutic doses most of the drugs producing haemolysis in G-6-PD deficient subjects have no effect in normal individuals, though dapsone is an exception and regularly produces mild haemolysis in most people.

Methaemoglobinaemia is produced by drugs and chemicals which increase the rate of auto-oxidation of haemoglobin. It occurs in normal individuals with large doses of the appropriate drugs, but is rapidly reversed by the enzyme methaemoglobin reductase, which is normally present in red cells, when the toxic agent is removed. In hereditary methaemoglobinaemia there is a deficiency of methaemoglobin reductase which is transmitted as an autosomal recessive trait, and homozygotes have spontaneous methaemoglobinaemia from birth. Heterozygotes have about 50 per cent of the normal enzyme activity and do not develop spontaneous methaemoglobinaemia. They are, however, likely to develop methaemoglobinaemia in response to drugs given in normal therapeutic doses and recovery is slow following removal of the drug.

Both G-6-PD deficiency and hereditary methaemoglobinaemia have a well defined genetic basis but some idiosyncratic reactions are only thought to have a genetic basis because they have occurred in close relatives. A well-known example is the irreversible aplastic anaemia which occurs in about 1 in 20,000 patients who receive chloramphenical. Chloramphenicol produces two types of bone marrow depression; a dose-related reversible suppression which is probably due to its effect on protein synthesis, and a rare aplastic anaemia. Aplastic anaemia has been observed in identical twins and evidence is accumulating to suggest that a genetically determined abnormality of DNA synthesis may be the underlying cause (Yunis, 1973).

Jaundice occasionally occurs in patients on oral contraceptives and may have a genetic basis. Two sisters have been described who both developed jaundice after taking norethisterone, a progestogen which is a common constituent of many oral contraceptive preparations.

Drug allergy

Allergic drug reactions are those which are produced by antigen-antibody reactions. They require sensitisation by previous exposure to the drug or a chemically related substance. Drugs vary greatly in their ability to act as antigens. Those with a high molecular weight such as proteins and peptide hormones can act as complete antigens, but most drugs are small molecules and become antigenic only after combining with body proteins. Some allergic reactions may be due to drug metabolites or to impurities in the preparation, rather than to the drug itself.

Drugs capable of producing an allergic response only do so in a few individuals. A genetic predisposition to allergy is probably required and atopic individuals are especially likely to develop drug allergies.

Sensitisation to a drug can be produced by any route of administration but is most likely to occur after topical use. Once sensitisation has occurred very small doses may produce a reaction and the clinical manifestations are determined by the antigen–antibody reaction and not by the chemical nature of the drug. Thus identical reactions are produced by different drugs, and the same drug may produce different reactions in different individuals.

Hypersensitivity reactions can be classified into four types, any of which can be produced by drugs:

Type I reactions. These are due to IgE or reaginic antibodies which are bound to the cell membrane of mast cells or circulating basophils. Combination of the antigen with the antibody releases histamine and other vasoactive amines. These reactions occur within minutes of re-exposure to the drug and the clinical manifestations are anaphylactic shock, bronchospasm, angioneurotic oedema and urticaria. They are most frequently produced by penicillin.

Type II reactions. In type II reactions the antigen is present on the surface of cells, and combination with antibody activates the complement system causing cell destruction. Many allergic blood dyscrasias are due to type II reactions: the drug forms an antigenic complex with the surface of the cell which is then destroyed by antibody. Examples are the haemolytic anaemia produced by stibophen, quinine and rifampicin; the thrombocytopenia due to apronal, thiazide diuretics and many other drugs; and agranulocytosis due to amidopyrine and phenylbutazone. The haemolytic anaemia produced by methyldopa differs from these in that it is due to autoantibodies directed against normal red cells and does not require the presence of the drug for cell destruction to occur.

Type III reactions. These are due to circulating antigen-antibody complexes which are deposited in the walls of small blood vessels producing an inflammatory response. The serum sickness syndrome is an example and occurs particularly with penicillin and the sulphonamides. Allergic pulmonary reactions such as that produced by nitrofurantoin are also of this type.

Type IV reactions. These are cell-mediated reactions due to antibody carried by lymphocytes. Contact dermatitis is the typical example and is due to external sensitisation to drugs like penicillin, sulphonamides, phenothiazines and local anaesthetics. Many exanthematous rashes and drug fever are also due to cell-mediated reactions.

It should be emphasised that this classification is an immunological one and more than one type of reaction may produce a particular clinical manifestation. Thus urticaria may be a type I reaction or may occur as part of the serum sickness syndrome. Also, although an allergic reaction probably underlies many drug reactions the precise mechanism is unknown. This is true of many drug rashes, of fever due to drugs, and of some types of drug-induced jaundice.

Long-term Effects

A causal relationship between an adverse effect and a drug is most easily established when the adverse effect occurs soon after administration of the drug. The longer the time interval the less likely it is that the responsible drug will be suspected, and if reactions appear some time after the drug has been stopped the relationship becomes even harder to establish.

Long term effects are particularly worrying because by their very nature they are often irreversible by the time they are detected, and because they include some of the more serious adverse effects of drugs such as carcinogenesis, blindness and chronic renal failure.

The precise mechanism of many long term effects is unknown and logical classification is impossible. However, they fall into two main groups:

(1) Cumulative overdose

(2) Delayed effects.

Cumulative overdose

Some drugs produce adverse effects only after prolonged treatment. These effects are usually dose-related, sometimes associated with deposition of the drug in the tissues, and may first become apparent or progress after the drug has been stopped.

Chloroquine is an antimalarial drug which has been used since 1965 in the treatment of rheumatoid arthritis. Large doses may be given for prolonged periods and elimination is very slow. The drug can be detected in the tissues for several years after stopping treatment and is deposited particularly in the pigment epithelium of the retina and in the corneal epithelium. The corneal deposits may cause blurring of vision, but they disappear when treatment is stopped. The retinopathy is more serious as it is usually progressive and leads eventually to irreversible loss of vision. Although visual loss may only become obvious after treatment has been stopped, it can be prevented by early detection of asymptomatic changes in retinal function.

The phenothiazines are also stored in retinal pigment cells and produce a retinopathy which, like that due to chloroquine, is related to dose and duration of therapy and may result in progressive visual deterioration after therapy has ceased.

Abuse of analgesic mixtures containing phenacetin, acetylsalicylic acid or amidopyrine is associated with a chronic interstitial nephritis and papillary necrosis which eventually produces chronic renal failure. The lesion appears to be related to the total amount of analgesic consumed and only occurs after prolonged heavy use, but the precise role of individual analgesics is not yet established. Analgesics are usually abused in combination and phenacetin is present in most of the combinations known to produce nephropathy. Acetylsalicylic acid is consumed in a much larger scale than phenacetin and prolonged salicylate therapy is often given in rheumatoid arthritis. However, there have been very few reports of analgesic nephropathy in patients taking salicylates alone. While salicylates and other analgesics such as paracetemol, amidopyrine and phenylbutazone may contribute to the development of analgesic nephropathy, epidemiological evidence strongly points to phenacetin being the main culprit.

The unwanted effects of prolonged treatment with pharmacological doses of corticosteroids are well-known and include osteoporosis, muscle wasting, skin atrophy and peptic ulceration. Prolonged suppression of the pituitary results in adrenal atrophy and an inability to increase steroid production in response to stress.

Long term alteration of normal endocrine function is also responsible for the amenorrhoea and infertility which sometimes follow prolonged use of oral contraceptives.

The long term effects of many drugs used in the treatment of chronic diseases are unknown and may first be noticed many years after the immediate adverse effects have been well documented. Extrapyramidal syndromes produced by the phenothiazines are well known and reversible on stopping treatment. Recently, however, a dyskinetic syndrome has been described which affects the tongue and facial muscles, occurs late in the course of treatment, and may persist after the drug has been stopped.

Delayed effects

Adverse effects which occur months or years after the use of a drug are rarely reported, but this may be due as much to the difficulty in establishing a causal relationship as to actual rarity of occurrence. The best-known delayed effect is the hypothyroidism which occurs following treatment of thyrotoxicosis with ^{131}I. The rate of onset of hypothyroidism is related to the dose of ^{131}I, but a dose which is sufficient to control thyrotoxicosis within a reasonable time without other treatment will almost inevitably result in hypothyroidism eventually.

Drug induced neoplasia is the most serious type of delayed effect; and one of the main purposes of preclinical toxicity testing is to detect possible carcinogenicity. The mechanisms whereby a drug may produce neoplasia are not well understood. For many carcinogens the affect appears to be dose related and neoplasms occur at the site of maximum concentration of the drug. Thus thorotrast which is concentrated in the reticulo-endothelial cells of the liver produces hepatic haemangioepitheliomas; carcinoma of the renal pelvis has been reported in association with analgesic nephropathy; and arsenic is deposited in the skin where it produces pigmentation, keratoses, and other skin lesions, which may be followed by the development of multiple basal cell carcinomata.

It is well known that exposure to radiation may cause leukaemia and as many cytotoxic drugs produce similar cell damage it might be expected that prolonged use could cause leukaemia. There have now been many reports of acute leukaemia following the treatment of multiple myeloma with melphalan, and a few cases have also been described following thiotepa and cyclophosphamide. The risk, however, is difficult to assess because these drugs are generally given for conditions which may themselves predispose to leukaemia.

Leukaemia may also follow damage to the bone marrow by other drugs. Several cases of acute leukaemia have been described in patients who have survived marrow hypoplasia due to chloramphenicol, and an association between acute leukaemia and previous consumption of phenylbutazone has also been reported though a causal relationship has not been established.

The growth of some tumours is hormone-dependent and there has been concern that prolonged use of oral contraceptives might predispose to carcinoma of the breast or cervix. This fear appears to be unfounded but in recent years an association has been described between adeno-carcinoma of the vagina in young females and the administration of high doses of stilboestrol to the mother in early pregnancy.

Finally, prolonged treatment with immunosuppressant drugs following renal transplantation appears to be associated with an increased incidence of malignant lymphomas in these patients, and it has been suggested that this may be due to suppression of immune mechanisms normally responsible for preventing neoplasia.

Conclusion

Although, to an extent which depends on their severity, adverse reactions limit the usefulness of drugs as therapeutic weapons, their identification may sometimes produce unexpected benefits. Often the search for alternative forms of therapy is intensified; drugs may be modified to increase specificity and reduce side effects, as was the case with the development of selective β-adrenergic stimulants; and completely new drugs may be introduced. Some unwanted effects may even prove useful therapeutically. Thus it was the observation of hypoglycaemia in malnourished patients on sulphonamides which led to the development of the sulphonylurea drugs as oral hypoglycaemic agents.

Adverse reactions have also been important in throwing light on disease processes, in revealing genetic differences and in studying mechanisms of drug action.

The number of drugs used in medical practise is now very large and the variety of adverse reactions that may occur is great. Some of these may mimic naturally-occurring diseases and produce diagnostic problems. The average doctor cannot possibly remember all these reactions, some of which occur very rarely, but he can and should remember always to enquire what drugs his patient has been having. He must have adequate sources of information about adverse reactions available, and he must remember to consult them.

CHAPTER III

FACTORS WHICH PREDISPOSE TO ADVERSE DRUG REACTIONS

To some extent unwanted effects are an unavoidable part of drug therapy. Those reactions which are not dose related are usually unpredictable and therefore unavoidable but it is possible to predict certain situations and identify certain patients in whom dose-related reactions are especially likely to occur. These reactions can then often be avoided (Table 3.1).

TABLE 3.1

FACTORS WHICH PREDISPOSE TO ADVERSE DRUG REACTIONS

Overdose
- Error
- During dose adjustment
- Cumulative

Relative Overdose
- Age
- Liver disease
- Renal disease
- Other disease
- Genetic variation

Overdose

The effects of gross overdose due to deliberate or accidental poisoning will not be discussed but lesser degrees of overdosage may occur for a number of reasons.

Error

The wrong dose of a drug may be prescribed or taken. In hospital this may be due to carelessness but it is especially likely to occur if prescription sheets are badly designed or if nurses copy out a "medicines list" and do not consult the original prescriptions when they administer drugs. The introduction of the "Aberdeen" type of prescription form has been shown to reduce these errors greatly (Crooks, Clark, Caie and Mawson, 1965; Crooks, Weir, Coull, McNab, Calder, Barnett and Caie, 1967). At home errors may occur because inadequate instructions have been given to a patient, but they are particularly likely to occur if a large number of medicines or tablets are prescribed, some to be taken once a day, others perhaps to be taken 2 or 3 times a day. This is a common problem with the elderly patient (Wade, 1972).

Less commonly the fault may lie with the manufacturer. There is increasing evidence that the formulation of preparations may modify the speed of absorption and the "bioavailability of drugs" (Smith, 1972). This is usually only of clinical importance where the dose of the drug administered to the patient is critical. In Australia in 1970 there were widespread reports of epileptic patients suffering from the toxic effects of phenytoin overdosage. The cause of this outbreak was eventually traced to an apparently minor change in the formulation of phenytoin tablets by the manufacturer. The reports ceased when the old method of manufacture was resumed. (Tyrer, 1970.) Recently there have been reports of wide differences in the bioavailability of different preparations of digoxin. A patient stabilised on an optimum dose of a brand with a low bioavailability of digoxin may develop signs of overdose when another brand is supplied to him in its place. This may happen when a patient leaves hospital or takes his prescription to a different pharmacist. In the future this problem will be solved when standards of bioavailability are laid down in the British Pharmacopoeia: for the present it is important with a few drugs for the doctor to indicate the specific brand of drug which is to be supplied to the patient. There is no need, however, for doctors to abandon the highly desirable practice of prescribing drugs by approved names just because this difficulty occurs with a small number of preparations. Anxieties about differences in bioavailability have been exaggerated to justify the use of brand names in prescribing.

Dose adjustment

Overdose can also occur during treatment with drugs for which the dose has to be carefully titrated against the therapeutic response. An excessive therapeutic response may occur if this is done with insufficient care, or if the patient's dose requirements fluctuate. A diabetic patient stabilised on insulin in hospital may develop hypoglycaemia when he leaves hospital and becomes more active, and a patient whose blood pressure is well-controlled while at rest in hospital may be incapacitated by postural hypotension when he has to get up in the morning on going home.

In the case of drugs with a low therapeutic ratio unacceptable side effects may appear at doses little above those required for treatment. If precise assessment of the therapeutic response is difficult, side effects are likely to occur while the optimum dose is being sought. This occurs commonly during digoxin therapy and in the treatment of epilepsy with anticonvulsants.

Cumulation

Cumulative overdose may occur with drugs which are slowly eliminated. If such drugs are given by repetitive dosing without a loading dose several days or even weeks are required to reach a steady state and toxicity may only develop at this stage. Digoxin therapy may be started with or without a loading dose. If no loading dose is given, at least seven days must elapse before steady state levels are achieved. If the dose selected is too large toxicity may only become apparent after the patient has left hospital. One of the arguments for giving a loading dose is that toxicity will occur earlier and the correct maintenance dose can be established sooner. In patients with impaired renal function cumulative toxicity may occur with any drug eliminated mainly by renal excretion if normal doses are given. This is discussed later. Cumulative overdose may also occur if a drug is concentrated in particular tissues. Thus chloroquine, given over a prolonged period, accumulates in the retina and produces retinal degeneration (p. 18, Chap. 2).

Relative Overdose

This occurs as a result of some abnormality in the patient. The abnormality may be one of drug elimination, impaired excretion or metabolism, resulting in an increased concentration of the drug at the site of action; or it may be an increased sensitivity of tissues to normal concentrations of the drug. Both drug elimination and tissue sensitivity may be affected by age, disease and genetically determined individual variation.

Drug interactions may also cause relative overdose. They are discussed in Chapter 4.

Age

Adverse effects of drugs on the fetus and neonate are discussed in Chapter 6. In the fetus they result mainly from the increased sensitivity of developing tissues, but in the neonate reduced renal clearance and immaturity of the hepatic enzymes that metabolise drugs are also important. Adverse effects involving the central nervous system occur more readily in infants and young children. Drug induced convulsions are more common and dystonic reactions to drugs such as metoclopramide are seen almost exclusively in children. Raised intracranial pressure produced by corticosteroids, nalidixic acid, tetracycline and vitamin A intoxication occurs mainly in children.

Elderly patients are also especially likely to develop adverse reactions to drugs (Table 3.2). Renal function declines with age and the elimination of drugs excreted mainly or entirely by the kidney is impaired. Thus adverse reactions to digoxin are common in the elderly and the aminoglycoside antibiotics, e.g. streptomycin, must be given in reduced dose to avoid toxicity. A small reduction in glomerular filtration rate may pass unnoticed or appear unimportant on routine tests of renal function yet be sufficient to delay the excretion of some drugs, and it is wise to assume a reduction when treating an elderly patient.

The ability to metabolise drugs is also reduced in elderly patients (O'Malley, Crooks, Duke and Stevenson, 1971) but the clinical importance of this has not been established.

TABLE 3.2

AGE AND DRUG REACTIONS

Age of Patients (Years)	No. Given Drugs	No. with Reactions	Rate per cent.
10–19	64	2	3·1
20–29	100	3	3·0
30–39	122	7	5·7
40–49	159	12	7·5
50–59	222	18	8·1
60–69	252	27	10·7
70–79	178	38	21·3
80–89	59	11	18·6
90–99	4	0	0
TOTAL	1,160	118	10·2

Rank correlation coefficient: y = +0·86

(Hurwitz, 1969)

Reduced tolerance to drugs in the elderly can also be due to the effects of age and disease on different organs particularly the brain and cardiovascular system. Drugs acting on the brain may have exaggerated or paradoxical effects; narcotic analgesics are likely to produce respiratory depression and hypotension, and sedatives may produce confusion and disorientation. Acute confusional states can be precipitated by a wide variety of drugs including the anti-parkinson drugs (benzhexol, 1-dopa), CNS depressants and digoxin. Homeostatic mechanisms are less efficient in the elderly and postural hypotension is a potential hazard not only with hypotensive drugs but also with many sedatives, hypnotics, tranquillisers, antidepressants and antiemetics.

Liver disease

Relatively few drugs used in man are excreted by the kidney unchanged. Most are first inactivated in the liver. Patients with liver disease may develop adverse reactions to drugs for two reasons: drug metabolism may be impaired or tissue sensitivity may be increased (Leading Article, 1973).

The effects of liver disease on drug metabolism are not well defined but in patients with severe liver cell damage the elimination of drugs metabolised by microsomal enzymes is impaired and this may lead to drug toxicity. Thus bone marrow depression produced by chloramphenicol is more common in patients with severe liver disease, and the increased sensitivity to sedatives and hypnotics may be partly due to slower breakdown of these drugs.

Patients with a history of hepatic encephalopathy or hepatic pre-coma may be extremely sensitive to the effects of narcotic analgesics, barbiturates and tranquillisers. Small doses produce characteristic changes in the EEG and larger doses may precipitate coma. This is mainly due to increased sensitivity of the brain though impaired metabolism may contribute. Hepatic encephalopathy may also occur if electrolyte disturbances are produced by diuretic therapy and hypokalaemia is particularly dangerous.

Hepatic synthesis of pseudocholinesterase, the enzyme responsible for inactivation of suxamethonium in plasma, is reduced in liver disease and prolonged apnoea may follow the use of this drug as a muscle relaxant in patients with impaired liver function. Reduced synthesis of vitamin K dependent clotting factors and a prolonged prothrombin time are common in severe liver disease and a small dose of an oral anticoagulant may produce haemorrhage.

Renal failure

Patients with renal failure may develop adverse reactions to those drugs which are excreted mainly or entirely by the kidney (Table 3.3). Even if a drug is inactivated by metabolism its metabolites may accumulate. These may be toxic (Table 3.4) or they may have pharmacological

TABLE 3.3

DRUGS EXCRETED BY THE KIDNEY WHICH PRODUCE ADVERSE EFFECTS IN RENAL FAILURE

Excessive Therapeutic Effect

Phenobarbitone
Chlorpropamide
Gallamine
Neostigmine

Increased Toxicity

Antibiotics — Streptomycin, Gentamycin, Neomycin, Kanamycin
Colistin and Polymixin B
Cephaloridine

Ethambutol
p–Aminosalicylic acid
Digoxin
Procainamide
Ethacrynic acid
Mercurial diuretics
Pentolinium
Lithium carbonate
Phenformin
Azathioprine
Methotrexate

TABLE 3.4

DRUGS PRODUCING ADVERSE EFFECTS IN RENAL FAILURE DUE TO ACCUMULATION OF TOXIC METABOLITES

Chloramphenicol	—	Bone marrow depression
Nitrofurantoin	—	Nausea, Vomiting Peripheral neuropathy
Nalidixic acid	—	Rashes, Photosensitivity Nausea, Vomiting

activity similar to the parent drug. For example the rate of elimination of amylobarbitone is not reduced in patients with renal failure but there is accumulation of the water-soluble metabolite, hydroxyamylobarbitone, which itself has some hypnotic effect (Balasubramaniam, Mawer, Pohl and Simons, 1972).

Drug concentrations may also be altered in renal failure as a result of changes in protein binding. Thus the protein binding of phenytoin in reduced in uraemia. Patients require smaller doses to achieve adequate therapeutic concentrations of free drug, and side effects are more likely to occur.

Some drug effects are particularly hazardous in renal failure. Drugs which cause vomiting, such as morphine, pethidine and some oral antibiotics, may produce dehydration with exacerbation of the uraemia. Tetracyclines and corticosteroids have a catabolic effect which will produce a

TABLE 3.5

DISEASES WHICH ALTER DRUG AVAILABILITY

Disease	*Adverse Effect*	*Drugs*
Hypoproteinaemia	Increased side effects of protein-bound drugs	Prednisone Phenytoin
Hypothyroidism	Increased sensitivity due to slower elimination	Digoxin
Heart failure	Increased risk of toxicity due to reduced hepatic clearance	Lignocaine

TABLE 3.6

DISEASES WHICH ALTER TISSUE SENSITIVITY

Disease	*Adverse Effect*	*Drugs likely to cause Adverse Reaction*
Respiratory failure	Coma precipitated by any respiratory depressant	All hypnotics, sedatives and narcotic analgesics
Myasthenia gravis	Increased sensitivity to drugs which block neuromuscular transmission.	Tubocurare, pancuronium, gallamine. Aminoglycoside antibiotics (streptomycin, etc.), Quinidine
Congestive cardiac failure	Aggravated by: (1) Drugs which produce fluid retention.	Cortiscosteroids Phenylbutazone Indomethacin Carbenoxolone
	(2) β-blockers	Propranolol Oxprenolol Practolol
Asthma	Bronchospasm produced	β-adrenergic blockers— Propranolol Oxprenolol Practolol (rarely)
Prostatic enlargement	Acute urinary retention	Diuretics Ephedrine Tricyclic antidepressants
Glandular fever	Increased incidence of rashes	Ampicillin.

rise in blood urea if renal function is poor. Patients with renal failure are unable to excrete potassium and may develop hyperkalaemia if given potassium salts or potassium-sparing diuretics such as spironolactone or amiloride.

Finally drugs which are nephrotoxic may exacerbate any pre-existing renal disease and should be avoided if possible. Many nephrotoxic drugs are excreted by the kidneys and are therefore, more likely to produce damage if renal function is already reduced. A list of nephrotoxic drugs is given in Appendix II.

Other diseases

Both drug availability and tissue sensitivity are affected by other diseases.

Tables 3.5 and 3.6 are not exhaustive lists, but contain some of the commoner examples for illustration.

Genetic variation

Genetic differences probably account for most of the individual variation in response to drugs and they play an important part in many adverse drug reactions.

In Chapter II some of the genetic abnormalities responsible for idiosyncratic drug reactions were described (Table 2.2). This section will discuss differences which predispose to adverse reactions by altering the concentration of drug available at the site of action or by altering tissue sensitivity. They can be divided into:

(1) Genetic differences affecting drug metabolism.

(2) Genetic differences affecting tissue sensitivity
   (a) Genetic variation in receptor sensitivity
   (b) Genetic disorders associated with increased sensitivity to certain drugs.

(3) Adverse reactions with an unexplained association with particular genetic traits.

Genetic variation in drug metabolism. The rate of drug metabolism is one of the factors which determines the concentration of drug available at the site of action.

Individuals differ in the rate at which they metabolise drugs and this is to some extent under genetic control. Two types of genetic variation are recognised: genetic polymorphism, where genetic differences are due to the action of a single gene: and polygenic variation, which is produced by several genes of small effect acting together. Genetic polymorphism gives rise to a discontinuous—usually bimodal—distribution (Fig. 3.1A) whereas polygenic inheritance gives rise to a normally distributed population (Fig. 3.1B).

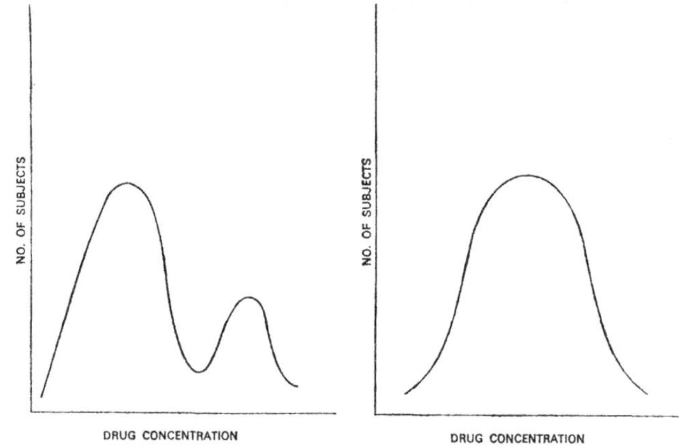

Fig. 3.1A (*left*) shows diagrammatically the plasma drug concentration found after similar doses of a drug had been given to a population of individuals with a biomodal distribution of fast and slow metabolic breakdown of the drug. Fig. 3.1B (*right*) shows a normal distribution of drug concentration after such dosage because the ability to metabolise the drug is of polygenic determination.

For many drugs which are metabolised by the non-specific hepatic microsomal enzymes variation in the rate of metabolism is normally distributed within the population and family studies have shown that this is partly under genetic control. Thus identical twins show close agreement in the rate at which they metabolise nortriptyline (Alexanderson, Evans and Sjoqvist, 1969), phenylbutazone, dicoumarol, antipyrine and alcohol (Vessell, Passananti, Greene

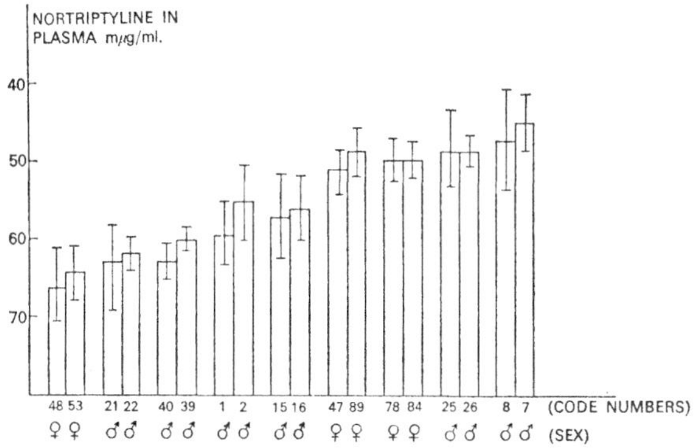

Fig. 3.2. Mean nortriptyline plasma concentration of days 6, 7 and 8 in identical twins previously not exposed to drugs. Data from Alexanderson et al. (1969).

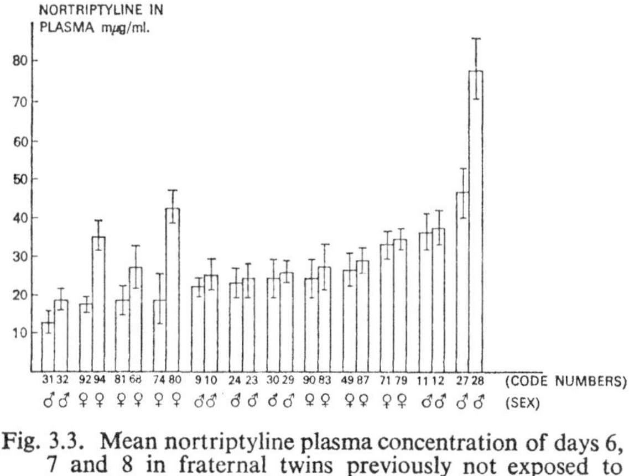

Fig. 3.3. Mean nortriptyline plasma concentration of days 6, 7 and 8 in fraternal twins previously not exposed to drugs. Data from Alexanderson et al. (1969).

and Page, 1971) whereas fraternal twins do not (Figs. 3.2 and 3.3). Furthermore, the normal distribution indicates that inheritance is polygenic.

Less commonly differences in the rate of metabolism of a drug have a bimodal distribution indicating control by a single gene. Isoniazid is inactivated by acetylation and the

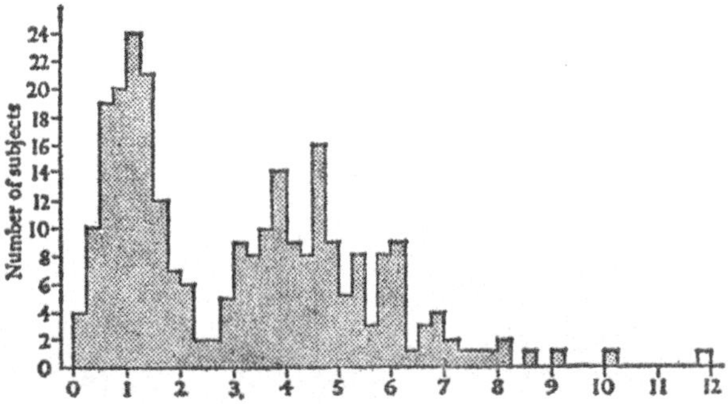

Fig. 3.4. Plasma concentration of Isoniazid (μg/ml.) 6h. following oral administration of 9·7 mg. per kg. of body weight in 267 family members of 53 families (Clarke, Evans, Harris and McConnell, 1968).

blood levels six hours after giving a standard dose to a group of individuals are bimodally distributed (Fig. 3.4). The population can be divided into slow acetylators and rapid acetylators, and family studies show that slow acetylation is inherited as an autosomal recessive trait. Other drugs inactivated by the same enzyme—N-acetyltransferase—include sulphadimidine, hydrallazine, phenelzine and dapsone, and they show a similar bimodal distribution of plasma levels.

A correlation between rate of metabolism and pharmacological effects has been shown for many drugs. Treatment may be ineffective if a drug is rapidly metabolised and dose related unwanted effects are more likely to occur in people who metabolise a drug slowly (Fig. 3.5). This will matter most for drugs with a low therapeutic ratio. Thus patients who metabolise coumarin anticoagulants slowly require only a small dose for adequate anticoagulation and may bleed if the usual dose is given. Patients who develop side effects from nortriptyline have a slower rate of metabolism and higher plasma concentrations than those without side effects. Slow acetylators of isoniazid have an increased risk of developing peripheral neuropathy—a side effect of isoniazid, and the incidence of antinuclear antibodies during treatment

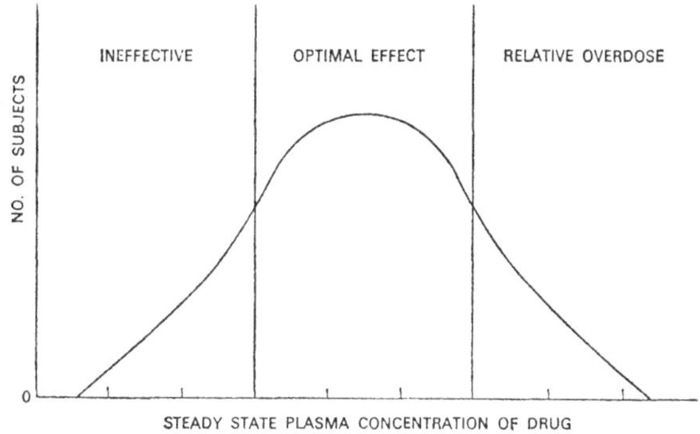

Fig. 3.5. A diagram that shows how, in a population, those who metabolise a drug very rapidly may have ineffective plasma levels of the drug and derive no benefit, while those who metabolise it very slowly may have very high plasma levels and suffer from adverse reactions.

with hydrallazine is higher in slow acetylators than in fast acetylators.

Another example of a pharmacogenetic polymorphism affecting drug metabolism is the rare suxamethonium sensitivity which occurs in individuals who are homozygous for an abnormal variant of the enzyme pseudocholinesterase. Suxamethonium is a short-acting muscle relaxant which is normally rapidly inactivated by plasma pseudocholinesterase, and suxamethonium sensitivity results in prolonged apnoea following its use during anaesthesia.

Both the acetyltransferase and the pseudocholinesterase polymorphisms show racial variation. The incidence of slow acetylation is about 60 per cent in Caucasians but only 10–15 per cent in orientals; and the incidence of suxamethonium sensitivity is higher in Alaskan Eskimos than in other races. Whether or not such differences are responsible for racial variation in the incidence of adverse reactions to other drugs is unknown.

Genetic differences affecting tissue sensitivity. Little is known about genetic variation in receptor sensitivity to drugs. Hereditary resistance to warfarin has been described in two families (O'Reilly and Aggeler, 1970), the members of which required very high doses and high plasma levels of warfarin to achieve an anticoagulant effect; and by analogy with warfarin resistance in rats this is thought to be due to a mutation in the vitamin K-warfarin receptor (Pool, O'Reilly, Schneiderman and Alexander, 1968). In any group of individuals there is a wide interindividual variation in the plasma level of warfarin required to produce the same degree of anticoagulant effect (Breckenridge and Orme, 1973), but although this may reflect differences in receptor sensitivity it has not yet been shown to be genetically determined.

There are, however, several inherited disorders in which the usual pharmacological effects of a drug are either exaggerated or potentially dangerous. Adverse reactions can usually be prevented from a knowledge of the nature of the disorder and the pharmacology of the drugs concerned. Table 3.7 gives some examples most of which are self-explanatory.

The hereditary hepatic porphyrias are disorders of porphyrin metabolism in which there is an overproduction of the enzyme aminolaevulinic acid (ALA) synthetase. Many drugs which are enzyme inducers further increase the production of this enzyme and may precipitate acute attacks of porphyria in patients with latent porphyria. Potentially harmful drugs are listed in Table 3.7.

Gilbert's disease and the Criglar Najjar syndrome are congenital abnormalities of bilirubin conjugation. In Gilbert's disease jaundice is mild or absent but can readily be produced by drugs which inhibit glucuronyl transferase (novobiocin) or which interfere with bilirubin uptake by the liver (rifampicin). The Criglar Najjar syndrome is a rare condition in which a deficiency of the enzyme glucuronyl transferase is inherited as an autosomal recessive. In the homozygous form jaundice is severe and commonly produces kernicterus. Heterozygotes have a less severe degree of jaundice but this is aggravated by novobiocin, oral contraceptives, and possibly by drugs which compete with bilirubin for conjugation.

TABLE 3.7

SOME GENETIC DISORDERS ASSOCIATED WITH INCREASED DRUG SENSITIVITY

Porphyria	Acute attacks precipitated by drugs which induce ALA synthetase	Barbiturates Meprobamate Glutethimide Dichloralphenazone Phenytoin Chlordiazepoxide Griseofulvin Sulphonamides Sulphonylureas Oestrogens and oral contraceptives
Unconjugated Hyperbilirubinaemia (Gilbert's disease Criglar-Najjar Syndrome)	Jaundice increased by drugs interfering with conjugation	Novobiocin Oral contraceptives?
Hypokalaemic Periodic Paralysis	Attacks induced by drugs producing hypokalaemia	Mineralocorticoids Insulin Carbenoxolone ? Diuretics
Primary Gout	Increased sensitivity to drugs producing hyperuricaemia	Thiazide diuretics, frusemide, ethacrynic acid
Haemophilia Von Willebrand's disease	Increased bleeding	Aspirin
Angle Closure Glaucoma	Increased intra-ocular pressure. Precipitation of acute glaucoma	Anticholinergic drugs—Atropine, tricyclic antidepressants, antiparkinson drugs Mydriatric eyedrops, e.g. atropine, homatropine, adrenaline
Sickle Cell Anaemia	Sickle cell crises due to anoxia.	Anaesthetics
Hypertrophic Obstructive Cardiomyopathy	Increased outflow obstruction	Digitalis

Adverse reactions with unexplained association with common genes. The ABO blood groups have been associated with a number of diseases, and recent studies of women taking oral contraceptives in the U.S.A., Great Britain and Sweden have shown a higher incidence of thromboembolic complications in those with blood groups A, B or AB than with group O. The reason for this is unknown though blood group O also appears to offer protection against thromboembolism in pregnancy (Lewis, Jick, Slone and Shapiro, 1971).

There is also epidemiological evidence that people with blood groups other than O have almost double the chance of developing arrhythmias when treated with digoxin (BCDSP, 1972).

Although such statistical associations provide further evidence that genetic factors are important in drug responses their clinical importance is likely to be small.

CHAPTER IV

DRUG INTERACTIONS

Recent surveys of drug use in hospital have shown that during their stay patients receive an average of 5–6 different drugs, many being prescribed simultaneously. Outside hospital fewer drugs are prescribed but self-medication with analgesics, laxatives, multivitamin preparations and proprietary remedies for minor symptoms is common.

Combinations of drugs are used for many reasons. They may be necessary if a patient has more than one disease or if different aspects of the same disease require different treatment. Drugs with the same therapeutic effect may be combined either to produce a greater effect than can be obtained with either alone or to obtain a greater therapeutic effect with fewer side effects by combining drugs with different side effects. One drug may be given to overcome the side effects of another as when atropine is given to overcome the side effects of neostigmine in the treatment of myasthenia gravis; or a drug may be given to prolong the effect of the primary drug by blocking excretion or metabolism as when probenecid is combined with a penicillin, or a dopa decarboxylase inhibitor with l-dopa. Thus many drug combinations are used to take advantage of specific interactions and there are possibly more interactions which are therapeutically useful than there are harmful ones. Drug interactions produce three types of unwanted effect: antagonism of one drug by another may result in loss of therapeutic effect; potentiation may increase toxicity or produce the effects of overdose; or an unusual reaction may occur which cannot be produced with either drug alone.

In this chapter the mechanisms by which drugs interact (Table 4.1) will be discussed with particular emphasis on the factors which determine the clinical importance of different types of interaction. Appendix III is a table of clinically important drug interactions.

TABLE 4.1

MECHANISMS OF DRUG INTERACTION

Outside the Body

- I.V. injections
- Infusion Fluids

Inside the Body

- Transport to site of Action—
  - Absorption
  - Protein Binding
  - Tissue Binding
  - Intracellular Transport
- Removal from site of Action—
  - Renal Excretion
  - Metabolism — Enzyme Induction
    Enzyme Inhibition
- Alteration of Effect of site of Action—
  - Competition at receptor sites
  - Interaction between drugs acting at same site or on same system
  - Alteration of Physiological Factors
- Mutual Toxicity

Outside the Body

Chemical or physical interactions frequently occur when drugs are mixed before administration. This is most likely to occur when drugs are added to intravenous infusions. The usual result is inactivation or precipitation of the drug with loss of therapeutic effect. A drug may be unstable in fluids used for intravenous infusions (Table 4.2), or it may interact with another drug added to the same infusion. A few important examples are given in Table 4.3 but there are many others and it is best to avoid mixing any drugs in intravenous infusions unless compatibility is well established.

TABLE 4.2

STABILITY OF DRUGS IN I.V. FLUIDS

Benzylpenicillin	Loses 10% of its activity in 4–8 hours in dextrose and dextrose/saline
Ampicillin	Loses 10% of its activity in 2–4 hours in dextrose and dextrose/saline
Methicillin	Loses 10% of its activity in 5–6 hours in dextrose, dextrose/saline, and saline
Gentamicin	Adequate serum levels may not be achieved if given by continuous infusion and it is best given intermittently
Amphotericin B	Must be given in dextrose solution of suitable pH. (See manufacturer's literature)
Heparin	Inactivated by dextrose
Frusemide	Precipitates in dextrose
Calcium salts	Precipitate in sodium bicarbonate

TABLE 4.3

DRUG INCOMPATIBILITIES IN I.V. FLUIDS

Drug	*Incompatible with*	*Reason*
The penicillins (Na^+ or K^+ salts of benzylpenicillin and the semi-synthetic penicillins).	Tetracyclines (as HCl).	Precipitation
	Gentamicin	Inactivation of gentamicin
Carbenicillin	Kanamycin	Inactivation of carbenicillin
	Colistin	Inactivation of colistin
	Gentamicin	Reduced activity of gentamicin

TABLE 4.3—*continued*

DRUG INCOMPATIBILITIES IN I.V. FLUIDS

Tetracyclines (HCl)	Penicillin	Precipitation
	Suplhonamides (Na+ salts)	Precipitation
	Hydrocortisone sodium succinate	Precipitation
	Calcium salts	Tetracycline chelate formed
	Sodium bicarbonate	Precipitation
Gentamicin	Ampicillin	Reduced activity of gentamicin
	Carbenicillin	Reduced activity of gentamicin
	Heparin sodium	Precipitation
	Cloxacillin	Precipitation
	Cephalothin	Precipitation
Heparin sodium	Aminoglycoside antibiotics (Gentamicin, kanamycin, streptomycin)	Precipitation
	Hydrocortisone sodium succinate	Precipitation
Hydrocortisone sodium succinate	Ampicillin	Inactivation
	Methicillin	Inactivation
	Tetracyclines (HCl)	Precipitation
	Heparin sodium	Precipitation
Calcium salts	Tetracyclines (HCl)	Tetracycline chelate formed
Phenothiazines e.g. chlorpromazine Barbiturates Phenytoin Vitamin B complex ± vitamin C Amphotericin B Sulphadimidine and sulphadiazine Frusemide	These should not be mixed with any other drugs in solution	

Inside the Body

Interactions occurring after administration may either alter the concentration of active drug at its site of action, or without altering its concentration may alter the response to the drug.

Interactions affecting Transport to Site of Action

Interactions affecting absorption

Drug interactions can affect either the rate of absorption or the total amount absorbed. In general, interactions which reduce the total amount absorbed will be the more important as the effect will be equivalent to giving a smaller dose. The rate of absorption is likely to matter most when a single dose of a drug is given to produce an immediate effect, e.g. an analgesic. It will be less important where a drug is given regularly to achieve a continuous effect as is the case with digoxin, antidepressants or anticoagulants. Drug interactions may alter absorption by a number of mechanisms:

Changes in gastric pH. Gastric pH affects drug absorption mainly by determining the rate at which a drug goes into solution from tablets or capsules (=dissolution rate). Basic drugs are more soluble in acid solution, acidic drugs in alkaline solution. Thus sodium bicarbonate increases the absorption of aspirin and decreases the absorption of tetracycline. Changes in gastric pH are probably not of great importance clinically.

Changes in gastrointestinal mobility. Drugs are absorbed mainly from the upper small intestine and the rate of gastric emptying would be expected to affect the rate of absorption. Food is known to delay the absorption of many drugs—probably by delaying gastric emptying—and drugs which affect gastric motility may influence the absorption of other drugs. Propantheline delays gastric emptying and has been shown to reduce the rate of absorption of paracetamol whereas metoclopramide which increases the rate of gastric emptying increases the rate of absorption of paracetamol (Nimmo, Heading, Tothill and Prescott, 1973). However, if a drug is poorly soluble rapid gastric emptying may reduce absorption by limiting the time available for dissolution, and this may be why the absorption of digoxin is reduced by metoclopramide and increased by propantheline (Manninen, Apajalahti, Melin and Karesoja, 1973). Rapid transit through the intestine, such as is produced by laxatives might reduce the total absorption of slowly absorbed drugs like digoxin, but evidence that this occurs clinically is lacking.

Chelation or binding of drugs. Drugs can interact in the lumen of the gut to form insoluble complexes which are not absorbed. Tetracycline forms complexes with divalent and trivalent cations and total absorption is reduced if it is given together with oral iron salts (Neuvonen, Gothoni, Hackman and Björksten, 1970) or antacids containing calcium, magnesium or aluminium. Cholestyramine, an anion exchange resin used in the treatment of hypercholesterolaemia, binds many acidic drugs in the gut lumen and reduces the absorption of both thyroxine and warfarin.

Most interactions modifying drug absorption can be avoided if the interacting drugs are given at different times —usually a 2 hour interval is sufficient—and are, therefore, not an absolute bar to concurrent administration provided they are anticipated.

Malabsorption syndromes. Both neomycin and p-aminosalicylic acid can produce a malabsorption syndrome and it is not surprising, therefore, that neomycin can reduce the absorption of phenoxymethylpenicillin, and p-aminosalicylic acid has been found to reduce the absorption of rifampicin (Boman, Hanngren, Malmborg, Borgo and Sjöqvist, 1971). *(*See* note on page 58.)

Protein binding

After absorption most drugs are carried in the bloodstream partly bound to plasma proteins. The degree of binding varies between drugs and binding is reversible, free drug being in equilibrium with bound drug. Only the free drug can diffuse out of the vascular compartment and exert a pharmacological effect, and it is the concentration of free drug which determines the rate of elimination of drugs which are metabolised by the liver or excreted unchanged by glomerular filtration. Protein-binding sites are non-specific and one drug can displace another from a site thereby increasing its concentration in the free form, increasing the availability at the site of its action, and increasing the rate of its elimination. The initial effect will be potentiation of the displaced drug but the duration of this will be limited by the increased rate of elimination and the final effect will be a return of the free concentration of the drug to previous levels with a fall in total plasma concentration.

Many drugs will displace each other from protein-binding in vitro but displacement will only be important in vivo if the following criteria are fulfilled:

(1) The displaced drug is highly protein bound. If a drug is more than 90 per cent. bound to protein, displacement of only a small amount will have a significant effect on the free concentration whereas if more than 50 per cent. is already free, a small increase will have little effect.

(2) The binding sites are easily saturated at normal therapeutic blood levels of the two drugs. Many acidic drugs (phenylbutazone, warfarin, aspirin, sulphonamides, tolbutamide) share binding sites which are readily saturated at therapeutic doses and important interactions can occur between them (Fig. 4.1). For the same reasons interactions are only likely to be important if the daily dose of the displacing drug exceeds several hundred milligrams. Both phenylbutazone and indomethacin are highly protein-bound and displace warfarin in vitro but the therapeutic blood level of phenylbutazone is greater than 100 μg per cent. whereas that of indomethacin is less than 2 μg per cent. In vivo phenylbutazone significantly potentiates warfarin while indomethacin has little effect.

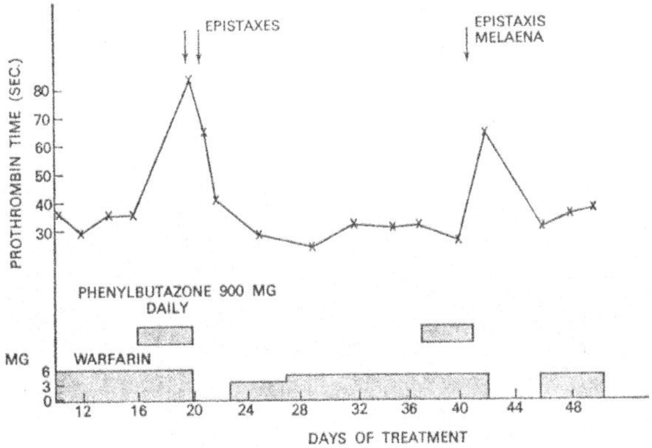

Fig. 4.1. The effect of phenylbutazone in a patient receiving warfarin. Phenylbutazone was given to treat acute gout and on two occasions resulted in an increased in prothrombin time associated with haemorrhage. (Beeley, L. — unpublished observations).

(3) The drug is not widely distributed throughout the body. Any drug displaced from protein binding will be distributed throughout the volume of distribution of the drug and the wider the distribution the smaller the absolute increase in the plasma concentration of free drug. Many basic drugs such as procainamide and the tricyclic antidepressants have a volume of distribution many times greater than the plasma volume. Thus, although they are highly protein-bound, displacement is not important clinically. Warfarin, on the other hand is not widely distributed and displacement from binding can be important.

(4) Even if an important amount of a drug is displaced the duration of the clinical potentiation will depend on the rate of drug elimination. The potentiation is likely to be important if the usual rate of elimination is slow or if the drug is eliminated by renal tubular secretion which is unaffected by changes in concentration of free drug.

In summary, displacement of drugs from protein-binding occurs commonly but important clinical consequences are much less common. Table 4.4 lists the interactions due to displacement which appear to have clinical importance. However, only the interactions between warfarin and phenylbutazone, and warfarin and chloral hydrate have been shown unequivocally to be due to displacement from protein binding.

TABLE 4.4

INTERACTIONS DUE TO DISPLACEMENT FROM PROTEIN BINDING

Drug Displaced	*Displacing Drug*
Warfarin	Phenylbutazone Oxyphenbutazone Chloral hydrate Clofibrate
Tolbutamide	Phenylbutazone Sulphaphenazole

Tissue binding

Although many drugs are bound to tissues, displacement of one drug by another is not known to be an important cause of drug interactions. It is possible that the increased toxicity of primaquine and pamaquine given to patients who have already received mepacrine in the treatment of malaria is due to reduced tissue binding of these drugs in the presence of mepacrine. However, this mechanism has not been established and mepacrine and pamaquine are now seldom used in the treatment of malaria.

Intracellular transport

Many drug interactions can occur at adrenergic nerve endings and sometimes one drug interferes with the uptake of another to its intracellular site of action. The antihypertensive drugs, guanethidine, bethanidine and debrisoquine are taken up by an active transport mechanism which is inhibited by some sympathomimetic amines and by the tricyclic antidepressants (Oates, Mitchell, Feagin, Kaufmann and Shand, 1971). The antihypertensive effect of these drugs is inhibited by therapeutic doses of most of the tricyclic antidepressants and by many common cold remedies which contain sympathomimetic amines such as ephedrine and phenylpropanolamine (Misage and McDonald, 1970).

TABLE 4.5

PROPRIETARY PREPARATIONS CONTAINING PHENYLPROPANOLAMINE

	Tablets or Capsules (mg)	*Syrup or Linctus* (mg per 5ml)
Mucron	32	—
Contac 400	50	—
Eskornade	50	15
Triominic	50	12·5
Triotussic	12·5	12·5
Triogesic	12·5	3
Runurel	25	25
Dimotapp	15	5
Dimotane	—	5
Tixylix	—	5
Vallex	—	10

Table 4.5 shows some of the proprietary preparations which contain sufficient phenylpropanolamine to inhibit the uptake of antihypertensive drugs. The tricyclic antidepressants also block the uptake of noradrenaline into adrenergic nerve terminals. This potentiates the pressor effect of noradrenaline given systematically since the main route of inactivation is by neuronal uptake. Severe hypertensive reactions have occurred in dentistry when local anaesthetics containing noradenaline have been used in patients being treated with a tricyclic antidepressant (Boakes, Laurence, Lovel, O'Neill and Verrill, 1972).

Interactions affecting Drug Elimination

Most drugs are removed from the body either by excretion of the unchanged drug in urine or bile, or by metabolism to inactive substances which are then excreted either in the urine or in the bile.

Renal excretion

Only water soluble drugs are excreted unchanged in the urine in significant amounts. Excretion is either by glomerular filtration or by active secretion across the proximal tubular epithelium. The excretion of weak acids and bases is pH dependant while the excretion of drugs by filtration depends also on the glomerular filtration rate and the extent to which the drug is protein-bound. Changes in urinary pH are not an important cause of drug interactions and little is known about the effects of drugs on glomerular filtration rate. Interactions involving displacement from protein-binding have already been discussed and may result in an increase in excretion by filtration. Many acidic drugs and drug metabolites are actively secreted across the proximal tubule. They share the same transport mechanism and compete with each other for secretion (Table 4.6). Interactions between some of these drugs may be clinically important. Probenecid delays the excretion of penicillins and this is used to advantage when high concentrations are

TABLE 4.6

SOME ACIDIC DRUGS THAT UNDERGO ACTIVE TUBULAR SECRETION

Probenecid
Sulphinpyrazone
Phenylbutazone, oxyphenbutazone
Indomethacin
Aspirin
Penicillins
p-Aminosalicylic acid
Dapsone
Dicoumarol
Methotrexate
Thiazide diuretics, frusemide, ethacrynic acid
Chlorpropamide

required; but probenecid also interferes with the excretion of dapsone, p-aminosalicyclic acid and indomethacin, cumulation of which may result in toxicity. Phenylbutazone interferes with secretion of chlorpropamide, an interaction which may produce dangerous hypoglycaemia (Thomsen, Ostenfeld and Kristensen, 1970). Other examples will be found in Appendix III. Organic bases also share a common pathway for tubular excretion but important interactions between them have not been described.

Drug metabolism

Lipid soluble drugs are inactivated by metabolism and excreted in the urine as water-soluble conjugates. Metabolism occurs mainly in the liver and most drugs are metabolised by the enzymes of the endoplastic reticulum (microsomal enzymes). Microsomal enzymes are relatively non-specific and can metabolise a wide variety of different drugs. Interactions between these drugs occur as a result of changes in the activity of the microsomal enzymes.

Enzyme induction. Microsomal drug metabolism can be accelerated by many drugs. This is associated with an increase in microsomal enzyme protein and is called "enzyme induction". More than 250 drugs are known to be enzyme inducers in animals but relatively few of these are important clinically (Table 4.7). Whether or not induction occurs depends not only on the nature of the drug but also on the dose used and the duration of treatment. Drugs used in a

TABLE 4.7

DRUGS WHICH PRODUCE SIGNIFICANT ENZYME INDUCTION IN MAN

Barbiturates
Glutethimide
Phenazone (as in dichloralphenazone)
Phenytoin
Carbamazepine
Alcohol (chronic, heavy drinking)
Griseofulvin
Rifampicin
Phenylbutazone

daily dose of less than several hundred milligrams do not produce significant induction and this is probably the reason why many drugs which are enzyme inducers in animals have little effect in man. Also as induction takes from one to three weeks to occur it will only be important where a drug is given for at least this length of time.

Enzyme induction reduces the concentration of drug at the site of action and results in inadequate treatment. If the dose of the affected drug is increased so that treatment is effective, toxicity may occur when the inducing drug is stopped. The most important examples of enzyme induction are the stimulation of warfarin metabolism produced by barbiturates and other hypnotics, and the increase in steroid metabolism produced by phenobarbitone and phenytoin (Appendix III).

Enzyme inhibition. If the metabolism of a drug is inhibited there is prolonged action of the drug and an increased risk of toxic effects. Relatively few drugs are known to inhibit microsomal enyzymes in man but several important interactions depend on this mechanism (Table 4.8).

TABLE 4.8

SOME DRUG INTERACTIONS INVOLVING MICROSOMAL ENZYME INHIBITION

Enzyme Inhibitors	*Drugs Affected*
Isoniazid Sulthiame	Phenytoin
Dicoumarol—	Phenytoin Tolbutamide Chlorpropamide (possibly)
Chloramphenicol—	Phenytoin Tolbutamide Chlorpropamide (possibly) Warfarin Dicoumarol
Phenylbutazone Sulphaphenazole	Tolbutamide
Alcohol (acute intoxication)	Warfarin

A few drugs are metabolised by specific enzymes other than those of the endoplastic reticulum, either in the liver or elsewhere in the body, and inhibition of these enzymes may also result in clinically important drug interactions (Table 4.9).

TABLE 4.9

INTERACTIONS INVOLVING INHIBITION OF NON-MICROSOMAL ENZYMES

Inhibitor	*Enzyme Inhibited*	*Drugs Potentiated*
Allopurinol	Xanthine oxidase	Mercaptopurine Azathioprine
Anticholinesterases (e.g. Ecothiopate iodide)	Pseudocholinesterase	Suxamethonium
Disulfiram Metronidazole	Aldehyde dehydrogenase	Alcohol
Monoamine oxidase inhibitors	Monoamine oxidase	Sympathomimetic amines (indirect ones only)

Interactions between the monoamine oxidase inhibitors and other drugs were among the first drug interactions to be studied in detail and many of them are still poorly understood. Only the hypertensive reactions which occur with foods containing tyramine or with other sympathomimetic amines are clearly related to inhibition of monoamine oxidase. Inhibition of intraneuronal monoamine oxidase results in the accumulation of large amounts of noradrenaline in adrenergic nerve terminals. This is released by indirectly-acting sympathomimetic amines, e.g. amphetamine, tyramine, phenylpropanoloamine, ephedrine—producing severe hypertension. Dietary tyramine is normally metabolised by monoamine oxidase in the gut wall, and the "cheese reactions" occurs because inhibition of the enzyme allows sufficient tyramine to be absorbed to produce a pressor response.

Interactions which alter Drug Effect at Site of Action

The use of combinations of drugs is a common feature of modern therapeutics. One reason for this is to take advantage of interactions between drugs affecting the same receptor site or physiological system. However, undesirable interactions also occur and although they are often predictable from a knowledge of pharmacology they are an important cause of adverse reactions.

Competition at specific receptor sites

Many drugs produce their pharmacological effect by competition with natural transmitter substances at receptor sites. Thus atropine prevents the autonomic effects of acetylcholine and propranolol blocks the action of catecholamines on β-adrenergic receptors. The effects of competitive inhibition can be overcome by increasing the concentration of the transmitter. Curare and suxamethonium both antagonise the effect of acetylcholine at skeletal neuromuscular junctions but whereas curare does so by simply blocking the receptors, suxamethonium is itself an 'agonist' and produces depolarisation as well as blocking acetylcholine. Thus anti-cholinesterases which increase the concentration of acetylcholine, will overcome the effect of curare but potentiate the effect of suxamethonium. Neostigmine is used therapeutically to reverse neuromuscular block produced by tubocurarine during anaesthesia, but the block produced by suxamethonium may be unexpectedly prolonged in a patient using ecothiopate iodide eyedrops for glaucoma.

Another example of this type of interaction is seen in the use of oral anticoagulants. These act by competitive inhibition of vitamin K in the hepatic synthesis of various clotting factors, and the effects of anticoagulant overdose can be overcome by giving vitamin K.

Unwanted interactions may occur when two drugs acting as competitive inhibitors at the same receptor site are used simultaneously. Thus the tricyclic antidepressants, phenothiazines, tranquillisers, anti-histamines and the anticholinergic drugs used for Parkinsonism are all inhibitors of the autonomic effects of acetylcholine, and produce atropine-like side effects—dry mouth, blurred vision, constipation, etc. This additive effect is often forgotten when an anticholinergic drug is given to prevent the extrapyramidal side effects of the phenothiazines, producing an increase in the severity of atropine-like side effects. It is probably also the explanation for the acute confusional reaction which sometimes occurs when patients on a tricyclic antidepressant are given anticholinergic drugs (Rogers, 1967).

Interactions between drugs acting on same physiological system.

Interactions which occur between drugs acting at the same site or on the same physiological system may result in either an increased or a reduced response. As with interactions at receptors, many are useful therapeutically but they may also be a cause of unwanted effects.

In the treatment of hypertension, drugs acting at different sites are frequently combined to obtain a synergic effect. Thus propranolol prevents the reflex tachycardia which would otherwise occur in response to the hypotension produced by a vasodilator such as hydrallazine; and the combination has a powerful hypotensive effect. However, it is often forgotten that many drugs produce vasodilation and postural hypotension as a side effect.. These include the sedatives, tranquillisers, anti-depressants, narcotic analgesics, anaesthetics and alcohol—any of which may cause severe hypotension in patients on antihypertensive drugs.

Many drugs produce CNS depression—either as part of their therapeutic effect, or as a side effect—and their effects are additive. This may be hazardous when alcohol is taken together with sedatives, antidepressants or antihistamines particularly if the patient drives or works with heavy machinery.

Antagonism between certain antibacterial drugs can be readily demonstrated in vitro but its clinical importance is less certain. Penicillins act by inhibiting the synthesis of the bacterial cell wall and are ineffective if cell growth is prevented by chloramphenicol or tetracycline. Although there have been few reports of this antagonism occurring in the treatment of bacterial meningitis, its clinical importance does not appear to be great.

Other examples of this type of interaction are the potentiation of tubocurarine by drugs with neuromuscular blocking activity such as the aminoglycoside antibiotics, quinidine and ether; and the severe bradycardia which may occur when digoxin is given together with reserpine or propranolol.

Alteration of physiological factors

The increase in digitalis toxicity by hypokalaemia is a well known hazard accompanying the use of diuretics, but it is perhaps less well known that other drugs cause potassium loss. Thus carbenoxolone, corticosteroids and prolonged laxative abuse may all increase digitalis toxicity. Drugs producing fluid retention such as phenylbutazone, indomethacin, carbenoxolone, oestrogens and corticosteroids antagonise diuretic therapy and may also reverse the effects of antihypertensive drugs. Conversely patients with sodium depletion due to excessive diuretic therapy are very sensitive to the hypotensive side effects of sedatives, etc.

Mutual Toxicity

It is not surprising that drug toxicity may be increased if drugs with similar toxic effects are used together. Thus the ototoxicity of the aminoglycoside antibiotics is enhanced by ethacrynic acid and frusemide, and combinations of nephrotoxic antibiotics are more likely to produce renal damage than when used singly.

Finally, many drug interactions cannot be fitted into the classification used in this chapter because the mechanism is unknown. Examples include the antagonism by pyridoxine of the therapeutic effect of l-dopa and the possible potentiation of the tricyclic antidepressants by thyroid hormones which has been reported in a few patients.

Conclusion

In spite of the large number of drug interactions which have been described, their clinical importance is often unknown. Undoubtedly some are important, and some are potentially fatal; but many more are of little importance clinically, either because they rarely occur at normal therapeutic doses or because the result is of little consequence.

In order to assess the likely importance of a potential drug interactions we need to know: (1) how often the interacting drugs are prescribed together, (2) whether the interaction is likely to occur under conditions of normal use of the drugs concerned, and (3) the possible consequences of the interaction.

An interaction between two drugs which are frequently used together is of more importance than one between drugs unlikely to be given to a patient at the same time. Thus the potentiation of mercaptopurine by allopurinol is important because allopurinal is used to prevent the urate nephropathy which may follow treatment of acute leukaemia. The interaction that occurs between the adrenergic neurone blocking drugs (guanethidine, bethanidine) and the sympathomimetic amines present in nasal decongestants is important because nasal stuffiness is a side effect of treatment with this group of antihypertensive drugs. Interactions involving drugs which can be bought without a prescription are especially important not only because these drugs are widely used but also because a doctor may be unaware that his patient is taking them. Thus interactions involving aspirin, common cold remedies, vitamin preparations, antacids and alcohol are important.

Several factors affect whether or not a potential interaction will occur in patients receiving therapeutic doses of a given combination. The importance of the therapeutic concentration of a drug has already been mentioned: for example many drugs which can be shown to stimulate drug metabolism in animals do not do so in man at concentrations achieved by the usual therapeutic dose. Duration of treatment is also important and drugs used as a single dose rarely produce detectable interactions. Thus paracetamol has been shown to potentiate warfarin if given in a dose of 3 grams daily for 2 weeks but as paracetamol is rarely used in this way the interaction is unlikely to occur clinically.

Some interactions will occur in almost all patients given the two drugs (potentiation of warfarin by phenylbutazone, enzyme induction by phenobarbitone, chelation of tetracycline by divalent cations), but many affect only a proportion of patients at risk. There are several possible reasons for this:

(1) Individual variation in rates of drug metabolism may affect interactions involving enzyme induction and inhibition. Thus the inhibition of phenytoin metabolism by isoniazid only produces a significant increase in plasma concentration of phenytoin in patients who are slow acetylators of isoniazid (Kutt, Brennen, Dehejia and Verebely, 1970).

(2) In the newborn and in the elderly in whom both metabolic capacity and renal function are relatively reduced, interactions involving drug elimination are more likely to be important.

(3) The presence of certain diseases may affect drug interactions just as it affects the response to individual drugs. Patients with renal failure are more likely to develop prolonged paralysis when given an aminoglycoside antibiotic together with tubocurarine; patients with severe liver disease are more sensitive to the anticoagulant effect of warfarin and are more likely to develop dangerous potentiation when given a drug which potentiates oral anticoagulants; and in patients with hypoalbuminaemia displacement of drugs from protein binding may occur more readily.

(4) Some interactions only occur in a small minority of patients at risk, for reasons which are unknown. Thus

one patient on a monoamine oxidase inhibitor may eat cheese with impunity but another will have a fatal cerebral haemorrhage.

Regardless of the frequency with which a particular interaction occurs, its clinical importance depends ultimately on the consequences. Interactions which alter the available concentration of a drug will matter most for drugs with a steep dose/response curve whose dose has to be adjusted within narrow limits to achieve the optimal therapeutic effect. Thus among the most important interactions are those affecting the oral anticoagulants, antihypertensive drugs and hypoglycaemic drugs, producing either loss of effect or an overdose. Where a drug has a low therapeutic index drug interactions easily produce toxicity, as is the case with interactions effecting cytotoxic drugs or anticonvulsants. The most important interactions of all are those which are potentially fatal.

* (Page 44. Recent evidence suggests that this is due to binding of rifampicin by the excipient present in PAS granules.)

CHAPTER V

ADVERSE REACTIONS IN DENTAL PRACTICE

A dental surgeon should always enquire not only about the health of his patient but also about any treatment he may be already receiving and any reactions to drugs which he may have suffered in the past. Patients often fail to mention treatment they have been receiving for a long period of time and they are particularly likely to conceal information about treatment they are receiving for mental illness.

In this chapter the adverse reactions of the drugs used by dental surgeons in their work are discussed first, and there is then a section on treatment which patients may be receiving for other illness which may cause difficulties for the dental surgeon or be of danger to the patient during the course of dental treatment. Table 5.1 is a list of drug reactions which may present initially to the dental surgeon because they affect the mouth or teeth.

TABLE 5.1

ADVERSE REACTIONS TO DRUGS PRESENTING AS DISEASES OF THE MOUTH

Stomatitis	Drugs causing aplastic anaemia or agranulocytosis (Appendix II), particularly: Cytotoxic drugs Gold Phenylbutazone Oxyphenbutazone Antithyroid drugs Chloramphenicol.
Stevens–Johnson Syndrome	Sulphonamides and co-trimoxazole Barbiturates (Appendix II).
Gingival Hyperplasia	Diphenylhydantoin.
Oral Thrush	Broad spectrum antibiotics—especially tetracyclines. Xerostomia due to anticholinergic drugs.

TABLE 5.1—*continued*

ADVERSE REACTIONS TO DRUGS PRESENTING AS DISEASES OF THE MOUTH

Teeth:	
Dental decay	Drugs with anticholinergic activity produce xerostomia which predisposes to dental decay and periodontal disease (Bahn, 1972). Phenothiazines Tricyclic antidepressants and monoamine oxidase inhibitors. Antiparkinson drugs Antihistamines Antihypertensives Antispasmodics. Diuretic therapy may have a similar effect.
Discolouration	Tetracyclines given during pregnancy or to children under 7 produce yellow discolouration and enamel hypoplasia. The latter predisposes to decay.

Drugs used in Dental Practice

Anti-bacterial agents

Penicillins. The only serious adverse reaction to penicillin is anaphylactic shock. This is most likely to occur following intravenous injection of benzylpenicillin and it may be fatal. Less severe manifestations of penicillin hypersensitivity are erythematous and urticarial rashes. Patients should always be asked about penicillin sensitivity and it is important to remember that cross-sensitivity occurs between benzylpenicillin and the semi-synthetic penicillins, e.g. ampicillin, cloxacillin. For most purposes either erythromycin or possibly cephaloridine will be a suitable alternative in patients who have previously reacted to penicillin.

Tetracyclines. Should not be used in pregnancy or in children under 7 because they are deposited in bones and teeth producing discoloration of the teeth.

Metronidazole. Patients given metronidazole in the treatment of Vincent's gingivitis should be warned about the possible effects of alcohol. Like disulfiram (antabuse), metronidazole inhibits the enzyme alcohol dehydrogenase and unpleasant reactions with flushing, tachycardia and hypotension may occur if alcohol is taken.

Analgesics

Aspirin may cause gastric erosions and bleeding. The risk is very small in relation to the enormous quantity of aspirin consumed, but aspirin-induced haematemesis may be fatal. Aspirin should not be given to patients with a history of peptic ulcer, or to patients on oral anticoagulants. Many compound analgesics contain aspirin, and there is no evidence that buffered aspirin preparations such as *Alka-Seltzer* are any less likely to produce gastric bleeding. Paracetamol is the safest alternative for these patients. Of the anti-inflammatory analgesics, phenylbutazone and oxyphenbutazone produce dangerous potentiation of oral anticoagulants but indomethacin does not appear to have this effect.

Sedatives

These are often prescribed for apprehensive patients before dental treatment. Small doses of phenobarbitone or amylobarbitone are sometimes used, but more often it will be a benzodiazepine such as chlordiazepoxide or diazepam. In older patients these drugs may produce hypotension and giddiness. In all patients the sedative effect is potentiated by alcohol and antihistamines. Patients should be warned about this and about the danger of driving after these drugs.

General anaesthetics

The hypotensive effect of anaesthetics may be particularly dangerous in the sitting position. Intravenous diazepam has a similar hypotensive effect and may be equally dangerous.

Local anaesthetics

Inadvertant injection into the systemic circulation may produce dangerous toxic effects. Cerebral stimulation may lead to convulsions, followed by respiratory depression; and myocardial depression produces hypotension.

Allergic reactions are not uncommon with some local anaesthetics but appear to be rare with lignocaine and prilocaine. Rashes, bronchospasm and anaphylaxis can all occur, and contact dermatitis may follow frequent handling of local anaesthetics by those using them. Topical use is particularly likely to produce sensitisation and severe swelling of the mouth.

Many local anaesthetic preparations contain noradrenaline or adrenaline as a vasoconstrictor, and enough can be absorbed to produce a systemic effect. The tachycardia and slight rise in blood pressure which result are unlikely to be important in healthy patients but more serious arrhythmias may occur in patients with heart disease. Tricyclic antidepressants and some antihypertensive drugs potentiate the effects of noradrenaline and adrenaline with potentially dangerous consequences (see p. 64). Felypressin does not affect the cardiovascular system and is a safe alternative in these patients.

Drug Therapy which may be a Hazard in Dental Surgery

Corticosteroids

Corticosteroids are used in the treatment of a wide variety of conditions, including rheumatoid arthritis, autoimmune diseases, asthma, skin diseases, and to prevent rejection of a kidney transplant. After prolonged treatment secondary adrenal failure occurs and cortisol secretion cannot be increased in response to stress. Profound hypotension may then occur during surgery and anaesthesia. Patients on long term steroids should have the dose doubled before, and for 24–48 hours after, minor surgery. Adrenal function is slow to recover after prolonged steroid therapy and patients who have had a course within the past year should also be covered—as should patients with Addison's disease receiving replacement therapy. Intravenous hydrocortisone should always be available in case oral cover is insufficient.

Insulin

In diabetic patients controlled by insulin minor dental procedures under local anaesthesia do not require any special precautions. It is important to ensure that the patient has not missed a meal beforehand as this may result in hypoglycaemia with sweating and tachycardia followed by confusion and eventually coma. In the early stages a glucose drink should be given, but intravenous glucose—20–100 ml. of 50 per cent. dextrose—will be required if coma occurs. If general anaesthesia is required diabetic patients on insulin should be admitted to hospital.

Oral anti-diabetic drugs

Diabetic patients on chlorpropamide or one of the other sulphonylurea drugs should not present any problems during dental treatment. However, the effect of these drugs is potentiated by phenylbutazone and by sulphaphenazole and hypoglycaemia may occur.

Anticoagulants

Patients receiving oral anticoagulants are more liable to bleed after extraction of teeth though capillary bleeding stops normally if the prothrombin time is not more than twice the control value. For elective dental extraction the dose of anticoagulants should be adjusted to this level beforehand (by the patient's own doctor). For emergency extractions the anticoagulant can be antagonised by vitamin K_1 but this should never be given to patients with prosthetic heart valves as adequate anticoagulation may be blocked for up to two weeks.

For extensive procedures the patient should be admitted to hospital where fresh frozen plasma can be given. This restores normal clotting time to cover the operation and the immediate post-operative period without compromising adequate coagulation subsequently. Many drugs interact with oral anticoagulants (see Appendix III). Paracetamol and codeine are safe analgesics but aspirin and phenylbutazone should not be given. Diazepam and chlordiazepoxide can be used but most other sedatives should be avoided.

Antihypertensive drugs

In patients receiving antihypertensive drugs the blood pressure may fall during anaesthesia. Dental treatment requiring general anaesthesia is best carried out in hospital where appropriate precautions can be taken.

Antihypertensive drugs which act by blocking transmission at adrenergic nerve endings or by depletion of noradrenaline increase the sensitivity of blood vessels to noradrenaline. This is most likely to occur with guanethidine and reserpine and patients may develop transient hypertension after local anaesthesia with preparations containing noradrenaline.

Antidepressants

Patients with depressive illness may be receiving a monoamine oxidase inhibitor (e.g. phenelzine, tranylcypromine), or a tricyclic antidepressant (e.g. imipramine, amitriptyline, nortriptyline).

Patients on monoamine oxidase inhibitors may develop severe reactions if given pethidine. They may also have a hypertensive crisis if given an indirectly-acting sympathomimetic amine (e.g. metaraminol, ephedrine). This is because, in the presence of a monoamine oxidase inhibitor, increased amounts of noradrenaline accumulate in sympathetic nerve endings and are released by indirect amines. Noradrenaline and adrenaline added to local anaesthetics are safe because they act directly on the receptors and are inactivated by uptake into the nerve terminals.

Tricyclic antidepressants on the other hand prevent this uptake and may potentiate the effects of noradrenaline and adrenaline in local anaesthetics producing severe hypertension or cardiac arrhythmias. Felypressin is a safe alternative (Boakes, Laurence, Teoh, Barar, Benedikter and Prichard, 1973).

Cytotoxic drugs and immunosuppressants

Bone marrow depression frequently occurs as a result of treatment with these drugs. Thrombocytopenia may produce prolonged bleeding after dental extraction, and neutropenia increases the risk of infection.

CHAPTER VI

DRUGS USED IN PREGNANCY, THE NEONATE AND LACTATION

Pregnancy

Drugs pass from the mother to the fetus across the placenta by passive diffusion, the extent of which depends on the concentration gradient and on the lipid-solubility of the drug. Lipid soluble drugs rapidly enter the fetus but even relatively insoluble drugs will cross the placenta if given in sufficient dose for long enough. The concept of a "placental barrier" is therefore only relative and almost any drug given to the mother during pregnancy may reach the fetus.

The adverse effects of a drug given during pregnancy will depend on the stage at which it is given.

First trimester

This is the period of rapid cell proliferation and organogenesis. In the very early stages teratogenic drugs have an all-or-none effect—the embryo is either killed or it develops normally. After the third week congenital malformations may be produced (=teratogenesis), and the most critical period seems to be between the third and the eighth weeks of pregnancy. If the abnormality is gross enough abortion will occur.

The Risk. Several factors make it difficult to establish the risk associated with the use of particular drugs in early pregnancy. Congenital malformations are common. They occur with an overall incidence of 1–2 per cent. and the cause in most cases is unknown. It is probable that drugs account for only a very small minority of these malformations. Nor even when suspected is it easy to determine with certainty that a drug is causing congenital malformations, for a drug with low-grade teratogenicity may produce an undetectable increase in the overall frequency of some already common congenital deformity. When an association is established between a particular drug and the risk of congenital malformation, it may be difficult to separate the effect of the drug from that of the condition for which it was given. Thus many large retrospective surveys (Speidel and Meadow, 1972; South, 1972; Lowe, 1973) have shown an increased risk of several of the commoner congenital malformations such as cleft lip and cleft palate in association with the use of anticonvulsants in early pregnancy but the small increase could be associated with the presence of the epilepsy itself. The problem is easier if the abnormality produced rarely occurs spontaneously or if a high percentage of women exposed to a drug have abnormal babies, but it may still take years before the association is recognised. Phocomelia is a rare type of malformation yet it took six years and many thousand deformed babies before its association with thalidomide was established and the drug withdrawn.

Very little is known about the mechanisms of teratogenicity and it is rarely possible to predict on pharmacological grounds, that a drug may cause congenital malformations. Prediction from animal studies is unreliable because of species differences, not only in sensitivity to different teratogens but also in rates and patterns of drug metabolism. Many drugs which produce congenital malformations in experimental animals have not been shown to be hazardous in man. Conversely rats and mice, until recently the animal species most widely used for testing drug toxicity, are relatively insensitive to the teratogenic effects of thalidomide —one of the most potent teratogens in man.

Relatively few drugs are proven teratogens in man; they include thalidomide and the antineoplastic drugs, especially folic acid antagonists. Others are suspected of being potential teratogens, mainly on the basis of epidemiological surveys showing an increased incidence of congenital abnormalities in association with a particular drug. These include the anticonvulsants, dexamphetamine (Nelson and Forfar, 1971) and ethionamide (Potworowska, 1966). Some drugs have been used widely enough to warrant the conclusion that, used in conventional dosage, they involve little or no teratogenic risk. However, for many drugs the evidence is conflicting and the possibility of producing a congenital malformation should be considered whenever a drug is given during the first trimester of pregnancy.

Second and third trimester

Structural development of most organs is completed in the first trimester and drugs given after this are unlikely to be teratogenic. Instead they may affect the growth and functional development of foetal tissues and organs. Thus the developing ear may be damaged by streptomycin; tetracyclines are deposited in growing bones and teeth; and antithyroid drugs may produce fetal goitre.

In late pregnancy the fetus may be more sensitive to the pharmacological effects of many drugs. Immaturity of the fetal liver results in a relative inability to synthesise vitamin K dependent clotting factors. Thus the coumarin anticoagulants may produce fetal haemorrhage even when the maternal prothrombin time is within a safe range; and significant hypoprothrombinaemia can also be produced by phenytoin and by large doses of salicylates. Immaturity of the fetal bone marrow may explain why thiazide diuretics occasionally produce thrombocytopenia in the fetus but not in the mother.

Sedatives, narcotic analgesics and anaesthetics given to the mother during labour may depress fetal respiration and this may persist after delivery, as a result of immaturity of the drug metabolising enzymes in the neonate.

Appendix IV is a table of drugs known or thought to produce unwanted effects in the fetus. It is not intended to be comprehensive and further information can be found in Ashton, 1971; Wilson, 1973; Meyler and Peck, 1972.

Drugs in the Neonate

In the first few weeks of life the renal clearance of drugs is relatively lower than in adults, the liver is deficient in drug metabolising enzymes, and the elimination of several drugs is impaired. The protein-binding capacity for drugs is lower than in adults and there is an increased sensitivity of immature tissues to some drug effects.

The newborn child, particularly if premature, is therefore more susceptible to certain adverse drug effects.

Kernicterus

This is due to the toxic effects of unconjugated bilirubin on the brain. Mild, transient unconjugated hyperbilirubinaemia is common in neonates due to a deficiency of hepatic glucuronyl transferase. Much of this bilirubin is bound to albumin and only the unbound moiety is free to cross the blood brain barrier.

Drugs may produce kernicterus either by increasing the total amount of unconjugated bilirubin, or by displacing it from protein binding. They fall into three groups (Table 6.1).

TABLE 6.1

DRUGS WHICH MAY PRODUCE KERNICTERUS

Drugs which compete with bilirubin for glucuronyl transferase.	Novobiocin
Drugs which produce haemolysis in neonates due to immaturity of the glucose-6-phosphate dehydrogenase enzyme system.	Nitrofurantoin Sulphonamides Primaquin Phenacetin p-Aminosalicylic acid Synthetic vitamin K analogues: (menadiol sodium diphosphate, menaphthone, acetomenaphthone).
Drugs which displace unconjugated bilirubin from albumin	Sulphonamides Novobiocin Aspirin Indomethacin Tolbutamide Water-soluable vitamin K analogues: (menadiol sodium diphosphate).

Haemolytic anaemia and methaemoglobinaemia

Enzyme deficiencies in immature red cells account for an increased susceptibility to haemolysis and methaemoglobinaemia. Haemolysis is due to immaturity of the glucose-6-phosphate dehydrogenase enzyme system and the drugs producing it are listed in Table 5.1. Nitrites, sulphonamides, phenacetin and local anaesthetics may all produce methaemoglobinaemia.

Haemorrhage

Haemorrhagic disease of the newborn occurs during the first few days of life and is due to immaturity of the liver resulting in impaired synthesis of the vitamin K dependant clotting factors. The neonatal liver is more sensitive to drugs which produce hypoprothrombinaemia. These include oral anticoagulants, large doses of aspirin and some anticonvulsants—particularly phenytoin and phenobarbitone; and haemorrhage may occur if they are given to the neonate or to the mother in late pregnancy.

Chloramphenicol

Deficiency of hepatic conjugating enzymes leads to accumulation and toxicity. This produces the "grey syndrome" consisting of circulatory and respiratory collapse which may be fatal.

Tetracyclines

These may produce permanent staining of the second dentition if given to neonates (Appendix IV).

Oxygen toxicity

Exposure of premature infants to a high concentration of oxygen (more than 35 per cent.) may lead to retrolental fibroplasia and blindness.

Drugs and Lactation

Drugs taken by a mother may be excreted in the breast-milk in amounts sufficient to produce a pharmacological effect (Knowles, 1965; Meyler and Peck, 1972). Information for many drugs is lacking but a list of those which may harm the child is given at the end of Appendix IV.

CHAPTER VII

PROBLEMS FOR THE PHARMACEUTICAL INDUSTRY BEFORE MARKETING A NEW DRUG

There is a story that at the first operation at which James Simpson of Edinburgh was to demonstrate the use of chloroform as an anaesthetic, the attendant dropped and broke the bottle. As there was no chloroform readily available the operation was started without anaesthesia but at almost the first stroke of the knife the patient died. If that death had occurred while chloroform was being administered, this "adverse reaction" might well have postponed the introduction of chloroform as an anaesthetic. Indeed, looking back into history it is surprising how often chance has aided the discovery or introduction of drugs, and it is tempting to suggest that, had the present day demands for animal toxicity studies and clinical trials been extant, a number of drugs now widely used might never have been marketed. As recently as 1938 after Dodds, Golberg, Lauson and Robinson had synthesised stilboestrol and shown that its oestrogenic potency exceeded that of normally occurring oestrogens, the new drug was in wide use within a few months in many countries for a whole variety of gynaecological conditions, for the most part with no proper evidence of its effectiveness and with as far as can be seen from published papers, no anxiety being expressed about carcinogenesis nor about its possible long term effects on reproductive functions.

The situation has changed radically since the thalidomide disaster in 1961. Now no pharmaceutical company would wish, nor would the governmental drug regulatory bodies which exist in so many countries allow a new drug to be marketed until evidence could be presented that its use in human patients was justified and that the benefits of its intended use were likely to outweigh any ill effects it might cause. The evidence demanded is obtained from studies of the action of the drug and its toxicity in animals and in man.

Animal Studies

Mice, rats, guinea pigs and hampsters are widely used for screening the pharmacological properties of newly synthesised chemicals and their toxic effects. Studies on dogs and primates are also needed but for economic reasons must be carried out on a much more restricted scale. Experience has shown that the pharmacodynamic studies in animals have a relatively high predictive value in man. Toxic effects may also be predicted from observations made in animals but in the present state of knowledge there are some important toxic effects in man which may not be revealed by animal studies. Without any doubt the best safeguard is that the investigation of a new drug should be in the hands of experienced men, skilled in the interpretation of the results and knowledgeable about the limitations of the extent to which work in animals can be applicable to man.

The procedures for studying toxicity fall into two groups. Those in which a single administration of a drug to an animal allows acute toxicity studies to be carried out, and those in which a drug is repeatedly administered to an animal in order to investigate chronic toxic effects, in a short term study of less than 3 months, a long term study of 3–6 months or over the whole remaining lifetime of the animal.

The choice of animal is often difficult. Usually an attempt is made to select animals which absorb, metabolise and excrete the drug in as similar a way as possible to man. Indeed it is widely accepted that at an early stage of the investigation of a new drug it is justifiable to carry out a few detailed studies of the absorption, metabolism and excretion of the drug in man—usually very small doses of isotope marked drug are used for this purpose—so that subsequent animal toxicity work may be planned to be as relevant as possible to the use of the drug in man.

Acute toxicity studies are usually done in at least three different animal species one of which is not a rodent. Animals of both sexes should be used. The drug is administered by several different routes and the several dose levels. spaced logarithmically, should span a range from that which causes no observable effect to that which kills nearly all animals. The aim is to define the lethal dose and the effects of the drug on important functions such as locomotion, behaviour and respiration. The cause of death often furnishes important information.

Repeated administration of a drug is expected to throw light on its cumulative toxicity, the development of tolerance to its actions and its capacity to induce enzymic activity which may modify the rate and even the route of its metabolism. Although biochemical measurements, pharmacodynamic studies and direct observations of the animals are extremely important, the histopathology of the tissues is still considered the most reliable and sensitive method of detecting the toxic effects of a drug. It is difficult in animal studies to detect toxic effects of a drug on vision and on hearing, and virtually impossible to predict whether sensitivity reactions will occur when the drug is given to man or what those reactions will be. It is difficult to predict from animal work whether a drug will interfere with sexual potency in man.

Carcinogenicity tests. Confident prediction either of carcinogenicity or of non-carcinogenicity is not possible on the basis of the chemical structure or pharmacological actions of drugs, but drugs which damage rapidly growing tissues or are related to chemical compounds which are carcinogenic must be specially suspect. Usually carcinogenicity tests are carried out in rats, mice and hampsters. The evidence that a drug is carcinogenic may be of several forms. It may cause an increased incidence of one or more tumours, benign or malignant, which are found in the control animals. It may not increase the incidence of these tumours but they may occur earlier in the life of animals given the drug. There may be tumours of a type not seen in control animals or an increase in the number of types of cancer seen in single animals.

Teratogenicity tests. The predictive value of teratogenic tests is still open to question. The value of animal screening is borne out by the fact that all drugs which have been established as teratogens in man can be shown to be teratogenic in rats, mice or rabbits. At present, however, no method of preliminary testing in animals can provide absolute assurance against the occurrence of teratological disaster when a drug is administered to a pregnant woman. The greatest protection is achieved if the investigations are carried out by workers with wide experience of toxicity studies, embryology and reproductive physiology. Even then it remains wise to avoid giving any drug to a woman during pregnancy unless she needs it to protect her health and well being.

Mutagenicity tests. In recent years there has been increasing concern that environmental chemicals including drugs may be a hazard to mankind by causing gene mutations or chromosomal aberrations either of which may be a factor in determining the occurrence of cancer or of other diseases in future generations. Shortage of man power and of specialised research facilities make it impossible to submit all drugs to comprehensive mutagenicity tests. Priority has to be given to drugs related to compounds that are likely to be carcinogenic or mutagenic, to those which inhibit oogenesis or spermatogenesis, inhibit immune responses, depress marrow activity or, especially important, are likely to be given over long periods of time to a child or a young adult. In vivo cytogenetic methods are used such as scoring translocations in meiotic preparations of mouse testis, examining chromosome abnormalities in early mammalian embryogenesis and detecting gene translocation by fertility tests in F1 offspring. There are a number of promising methods under current investigation including fluorescent chromosome analysis, pachytene mapping and assay of body fluids for substances mutagenic to micro-organisms or other indicator systems.

Human Studies

Early investigation of a drug in man

Although, as stated earlier, a single administration of a small dose of a new drug to man may be justifiable after only a few weeks of animal toxicity studies to guide further animal work, it is seldom justifiable to administer a new drug to man in repeated doses until chronic toxicity studies of 3–6 months have been completed in animals; and sometimes it is wise to have completed lifelong animal studies.

The earliest use of a new drug in man is usually carried out in a small number of subjects under close clinical and laboratory supervision.

The main purpose of these early investigations is to determine whether the drug has a pharmacological action likely to be useful, and the dose needed to produce these effects. In general the preliminary animal work is reliable in predicting the effects a drug will have in man but does not indicate the dose at which they will occur.

The procedures which are appropriate in testing new drugs vary widely, being different for instance if the drug is a general anaesthetic, an antimicrobial, a cytotoxic agent or a dermatological preparation; moreover facilities, attitudes and legal restrictions vary from country to country. What is always important however is that there must be the closest co-operation between those who have studied the actions and toxic effects of the drug in animals and those who carry out the initial studies in man for sometimes it will be imperative to delay or interrupt the clinical programme while further animal work is done.

Depending on the nature of the drug, these investigations may be carried out on volunteer healthy subjects, volunteers with a disease not under investigation, volunteers with the disease for which the drug is to be used and sometimes patients who are resistant to current therapy. This last group may have to be used at the outset of investigations but a useful drug may be lost if it is given up after failing to help patients who have already failed to respond to existing drugs for such patients may suffer from unusual forms of a disease.

It is generally thought that this phase of the investigation of a new drug when it is being given to human beings for the first time is the time of greatest anxiety for those who are responsible for the work. This is true but in fact this phase is probably one of the safest for the investigations are done in a small number of subjects under the close observation of competent and well informed physicians and scientists.

Later studies in man

Although the early clinical studies may confirm that the desired pharmacological actions occur in man, much more extensive investigation is required to determine whether the therapeutic value of a drug is such that it is justifiable to market it. These investigations can never start until the long term animal toxicity rests have been completed.

Usually the purpose of these investigations, and they may be continued over many years after the drug is marketed, is to compare the new form of therapy with that which already exists whether it is drug therapy, surgery, psychotherapy or, perhaps, no therapy at all.

In Britain we are fortunate. It is widely accepted that properly planned clinical trials are the most effective method we have at our disposal to determine whether a newly introduced drug is or is not more effective than existing therapy. The trials of the new antituberculosis drugs carried out under the aegis of Sir Austin Bradford Hill between 1946 and 1952 (Daniels, M. and Hill, A.B., 1952) showed convincingly that a well planned trial in a relatively small number of patients could give information in a short period of time of a reliability which can never be attained by the casual use of a new remedy. The only exception to this is in the unusual circumstances when drugs such as the first sulphonamide of the first antibiotic make a dramatic impact on diseases for which there is no adequate existing therapy.

There is now an extensive body of knowledge and experience about the planning and the interpretation of controlled therapeutic trials. They constitute a most important tool in the evaluation of the effectiveness of new drug therapy but like most tools require competent and experienced users.

Clinical trials, as was the case in the classical trials of the anti-tuberculosis drugs, often have to be carried out at more than one centre so that sufficient patients can be admitted to the trial and treated in a relatively short time. It is especially important to define accurately the type of patient who is to be admitted to the trial, the way in which treatments are to be allocated and the criteria by which effectiveness is to be assessed.

It is not always appreciated that even when the desired pharmacological action of a drug has been confirmed and characterised its value to patients may be in doubt for many years.

There is for instance no doubt that a number of drugs, including clofibrate, can reduce the plasma levels of lipids: what is still uncertain is whether such drugs give worthwhile protection to patients who have already had a myocardial infarct or whether their administration to healthy persons as a prophylactic measure to reduce the incidence of coronary arterial disease is justified. What is certain is that if these drugs are shown to offer protection, extensive evidence of their safety will have to be obtained as rapidly as possible for unless this is ensured their use on a wide scale in healthy persons will be difficult to justify. Moreover medicine will be faced with new problems if men who are healthy are to be persuaded to accept long continued use of a drug to protect themselves against a hazard which is so unpredictable in a given individual.

Ethical problems of drug studies in man

There are a number of difficult ethical problems which arise when new drugs are first administered to man or when trials of drugs are carried out.

Children. In general everyone agrees that new drugs should be tested in adults, but some diseases do not occur or are not common in adults. New therapy for certain tumours, leukaemias, some genetic errors of metabolism or intended to protect against certain infections such as measles or whooping cough can only be tested in children. In our experience there is seldom difficulty for the diseases are serious and the parents are anxious to co-operate to find better therapy or protection. It is a field where the integrity of the investigator has to be of the highest quality to justify the trust of the parents.

Women of the child bearing age or who are pregnant should seldom be used for the early clinical studies of drugs. It is impossible to be dogmatic even about this as new therapeutic measures to prevent miscarriage or to treat diseases of pregnancy such as eclampsia need to be assessed.

Mortally ill patients. It is not only morally repugnant but also unwise to conduct early clinical studies of a new drug in patients who are near to death, for the effects of the drug whether good or bad are likely to be masked by the effects of disease and when death occurs the blame may be laid on the drug rather than on the disease.

Dependent subjects. Special care is required if students, soldiers, employees or prisoners are asked to "volunteer". They may acquiesce not because they wish to but because they believe that they may suffer in some way if they do not volunteer. Having said that, it is important to appreciate that what is considered quite unacceptable in one community may be looked on as normal and appropriate in another country or in different circumstances.

In the United States of America, when Dr. J. A. Shannon was asked urgently to carry out studies of antimalarial drugs at a time of national emergency during the 1939–1945 war when the world's supply of quinine had been lost to the Japanese in the Dutch East Indies, the prison inmates who were asked to volunteer as subjects to be infected with malarial parasites knew exactly what they were submitting themselves to and regarded volunteering as a personal contribution to their nation at war. Dr. Shannon and his colleagues thanked them in their paper for their enthusiastic co-operation.

In America there is now a long tradition of prisoners co-operating in research and there has been no anxiety that any exploitation of these volunteers has occurred. In Britain such work would not be acceptable.

Informed consent. It is widely accepted that patients or volunteers should be fully informed about the work, the drug and any risks to which they may be exposed, so that they give informed consent. This is not always easy to ensure: not all patients can understand the best intended efforts of explanation and indeed some may be made unnecessarily apprehensive about some very minor procedure. Moreover there are times when it may not be in the best interest of a patient to give full information. A physician may for instance feel it would be unwise to reveal to a patient that he is suffering from a relentlessly advancing neurological disease or cancer. Sometimes it is impossible to give any information to patients with mental retardation or mental illness who may be incapable of understanding explanations or giving consent, yet this is an area where new and effective therapy is badly needed. There are also times when revealing the full nature of the test may destroy the validity of the results of investigation. This is especially likely to be the case when it is necessary to determine whether the benefit supposed to be derived from therapy is due to suggestion rather than to any pharmacological action of a drug. In all studies carried out in patients or volunteers it is wise for the investigator to safeguard the patient's interests by consulting the views of a group of independent physicians and scientists, but this is especially important in any situation in which full informed consent cannot or will not be obtained.

Rewards. Any system of reward must be such that there can be no question of subjects being bribed to submit to unreasonable hazards. On the other hand, it is unreasonable to ask subjects to give up a whole day and perhaps a night during which blood and urine samples are taken at carefully timed intervals, without offering some compensation.

Similarly, it is highly desirable that those who plan and conduct clinical drug research should not have their judgement in any way perverted by excessive rewards. It is necessary to pay professional staff, doctors, nurses and technicians at standard rates of remuneration for work they do, but payment should not in any way depend on a "successful outcome" of their study.

The Supervision of Studies in Animals and Man

As long as there continues to be a need for new or more effective therapy for disease, the development and testing of new drugs must continue. The work in both animals and man demands the highest scientific and ethical standards. In Britain a Royal Commission reported in 1874 "on the practice of subjecting live animals to experiments for scientific purposes" and the rather unfortunately named "Cruelty to Animals Act" was passed in 1876. Since that time anyone who does experimental work on animals must be licensed by the Home Office and their laboratories and records may be examined at any time by Inspectors. The system is a good one. No professional research worker would ever risk the loss of his licence by carrying out studies which had not been approved by the inspectorate and despite intemperate claims by antivivisectionists animal experiments are not done unless they are necessary.

The standard of kindness and care in the handling of animals is very high and the inspectorate has made a major contribution by encouraging high standards of construction, hygiene and ventilation of animal houses.

The proper planning and execution of studies on new drugs in man whether in healthy volunteers or in patients is even more demanding. There has to be close co-operation between those who have developed the drug in the pharmaceutical industry and doctors who are responsible for the studies in man. Whether such work is done in hospital or in general practice all are aware that behaviour that was in any way unethical or unjustifiable or which did not put the care of the individual patient before the requirements of investigational work, would immediately be censured by medical colleagues.

As a result of the Nuremburg trials of those who carried out disgraceful and inhumane experiments on Jews and other prisoners in Germany between 1939 and 1945, the World Health Assembly meeting in Helsinki in 1953 promulgated a code of ethical behaviour to be observed by all who carry out investigation in man: it is known as the Helsinki Declaration. This Declaration and other codes of behaviour, regulations and laws are of undoubted value in promoting high standards of ethical behaviour in work on man. But experience suggests that the greatest safeguard is the wide acceptance by research workers that the purpose, plan and design of all research in volunteers or patients must be reviewed by independent medical ethical committees. These are more effective in protecting both the patient and the investigator than any law. In our country wise advice about the establishment of such committees, their composition and their terms of reference has been given by the Royal College of Physicians of London (1973).

CHAPTER VIII

MONITORING ADVERSE REACTIONS TO DRUGS AND THE THERAPEUTIC AUDIT

Monitoring the use of a drug after it has been marketed to identify and characterise any adverse reactions which it may cause is needed for two reasons.

Firstly, adverse reactions even if infrequent may cause serious morbidity and mortality to patients. Amongst the more serious reactions are anaphylactic shock, jaundice, blood dyscrasias and exfoliative dermatitis. Moreover, once a drug is marketed its use may rapidly become widespread and may not be confined to one country: the number of patients put at risk may be large.

Secondly, unless an active attempt is made to look for and identify adverse reactions they may pass unnoticed for many years. Aspirin was first used in clinical medicine in 1899 but the hazard of gastric erosion was not recognised until 1938. Cincophen was introduced as an analgesic of special value in gout in 1908, but the first reports of liver damage were not published until 1923. The oral contraceptives were introduced in 1957 but proof that they caused a slightly increased hazard of venous thrombosis and embolism was not obtained until 1965.

The purpose of monitoring

This has never been better stated than in a report on "The assessment of drug toxicity" prepared for the Medical Research Council (1963) which profoundly influenced the views of the Committee on Safety of Drugs and later the Medicines Commission. It stated "The purpose of determining the toxic effects (of a drug) in man will usually be to obtain intelligent restriction of its further use. To make such a decision possible it is necessary not only to recognise the toxic effect but also to estimate its incidence and determine the factors which increase the risk of toxicity." Ideally the risk of using a drug needs to be assessed in relation to the hazards of the diseases for which it is used and the efficacy of the drug.

Therapeutic efficacy is generally assessed by clinical trials and some estimate of the incidence of pharmacological side effects should be ascertainable at this stage. These side effects are usually predictable and rarely serious, but they may be sufficiently unpleasant to limit the clinical usefulness of the drug.

Toxic side effects that are not related to the known pharmacology of the drug are more likely to be unpredictable, may be serious but probably occur in only a small proportion of patients. Similarly adverse reactions which are not dose related may be serious and may be difficult to predict. The purpose of monitoring is to detect reactions of these last two types to define their incidence and to determine any predisposing or precipitating factors.

Spontaneous monitoring systems

The commonest form of monitoring developed in the last ten years in a number of countries has been the formation of registries of adverse reactions to which doctors and dental surgeons are encouraged to report suspected adverse reactions which they observe. To be effective these registries require cooperation from doctors but it is well established that only a tiny proportion of all suspected reactions are ever reported. In 1966 when the relationship between oral contraceptives and venous thrombosis was a matter of great public concern in Britain, all doctors were asked to report deaths due to thromboembolism in women using oral contraceptives to the Committee on Safety of Drugs. Yet when an enquiry was later conducted by officers of the Committee it was found that in a sample of 53 women identified by the Registrar General who had died of thromboembolism and who were known by their family doctor to be on oral contraceptives, only 8 (15 per cent.) had been reported to the Committee and only 2 of these 8 by the family doctor.

The most successful registries are in Britain, Sweden, Australia, New Zealand and Canada. The standard of the reports received in these countries has been high and the information useful and reliable. But even in Sweden where there is a legal duty laid on doctors to report adverse reactions to drugs, reporting is only a little better than in Britain.

In the United States of America reporting has been poor: this has been blamed on the high level of litigation against doctors encouraged by their legal system. Understandably a doctor is not anxious to put his name to a statement which makes it clear that he thinks his patient was harmed by a medicament that he prescribed.

However, despite these defects, spontaneous reporting systems are still the most informative of all systems in current use. It is believed that they could be made much more informative if the interest of doctors in adverse reactions to drugs could be stimulated. One way of increasing this interest is for the registry to feed information back to the medical profession about the reports which are received. In Sweden there is a quarterly bulletin sent to all practitioners and in Britain any doctor who reports a suspected reaction is sent a personal letter with details of all other reports about the drug.

Attempts have recently been made to increase the interest of hospital doctors by the appointment of Drug Safety Officers: these are usually medical officers but in Scotland and in the Midlands pharmacists and doctors have co-operated in this work. In the Midlands an Adverse Reactions Study Group has been established so that those interested in adverse reactions may meet together regularly and undertake studies of individual drugs.

Intensive surveillance

In the mid 1960's a number of studies were undertaken in which patients in hospital have been kept under surveillance, all drugs given to them and any suspected adverse reactions being reported. These surveys in the U.S.A. (Seidl, Thornton,

Smith and Cluff, 1966), Canada (Hoddinott, Gowdey, Coulter and Parker, 1967) and Northern Ireland (Hurwitz and Wade, 1969) all showed that the incidence of adverse reactions to drugs was greater than had been suspected. About 5 per cent. of admissions to medical wards were due to adverse reactions and 10 per cent. of the patients admitted to medical wards suffered from adverse reactions during their treatment in the ward.

The early pilot surveys have been followed by a major on-going survey at Boston, U.S.A. with the collaboration of hospitals in at least 6 other cities, not all of which are in the U.S.A. Although this survey makes it possible to measure the incidence of adverse reactions in relation to the use of a drug and to detect reactions due to the interaction of drugs, the returns have not in the opinion of many justified the cost, for it is demanding of staff. It would seem likely that smaller and less ambitious schemes might give a better return, possibly by concentrating on certain types of patients, on certain drugs or on investigations which might throw light on the mechanism of drug reactions.

Record linkage

It is difficult to detect and measure the incidence of adverse reactions that occur months or even years after the administration of a drug unless it is possible to assemble easily and and rapidly the medical records of a patient from a number of different sources from which he has received medical care, his family doctor, hospitals which he has attended or to which he has been admitted and clinics where he has been vaccinated. Eventually details of his death must be obtained from the Registrar General. A record linkage scheme which aims at doing this has already been started in Oxford and is planned in Northern Ireland and Scotland. There is little experience as yet to draw upon but it may one day be possible to determine whether the long continued use of drugs such as the oral contraceptive increases, decreases or has no effect on the incidence of malignant growths, whether the administration of a vaccine may in certain individuals adversely modify the nature of some illness acquired in later life or whether the administration of a drug in early life interferes with the use of the same or other drugs years later.

International cooperation

The World Health Organisation (WHO) has interested the health authorities of an increasing number of countries in the problems of adverse reactions to drugs and has created a forum for workers to discuss monitoring. The WHO Pilot Drug Monitoring Project made an important contribution by defining terms, making a dictionary of adverse reactions and devising codes for reactions, drugs and the chemical formulae of drugs so that information about adverse reactions may be recorded in an accessible form in electronic data processing equipment.

By enabling workers in the field to meet regularly a camaraderie has grown which has borne fruit: workers in the national centres now find that help, advice and information is always readily available, either direct from WHO or more often from colleagues in other centres. Originally it was hoped that information about adverse reactions from all the national centres would be collected together at WHO and that this would aid the identification and characterisation of adverse reactions which occurred so infrequently that no single country on its own could do it. Although a splendid concept, in practice this has not been very valuable. But the exchange of information on decisions made in different countries about restrictions of the use of drugs because of adverse reactions has been most valuable.

The need for a therapeutic audit

A criticism of present day work in the field of adverse reactions to drugs is that it has been too narrowly based, concentrating on the detection of previously unsuspected adverse reactions. Although this is important it is only a part of what needs to be done. What should be aimed at is a far more comprehensive "therapeutic audit" which identifies what drugs are used in a community, who prescribes them, to which patients, for what diseases or symptoms and with what results in terms of effective therapy which may or may not be marred by the occurrence of adverse reactions. We are a long way from achieving such an ambitious aim but some studies of the use of drugs have already shown that there are marked differences in the prescribing habits of different doctors, that changes in the pattern of prescribing are occurring all the time, especially when new preparations are marketed, that there are differences in drug use in different areas within a country and bigger differences between countries. All these need to be examined if the incidence of adverse reactions to drugs is to be seen in its correct perspective.

Differences between doctors

The broad spectrum antibiotic chloramphenicol was first marketed in 1949 and its infrequent but often fatal complication, aplastic anaemia, was first recognised in 1951. Over the next decade it was frequently discussed in the world's medical journals. The prescribing of chloramphenicol by doctors in general practice in Northern Ireland was investigated in 1962 and 1964 (Wade, 1966). It was surprising to find that in December 1962 there were 3,123 prescriptions written for chloramphenicol, 1,141 for capsules and 1,982 for syrup, probably mainly for children. Yet of the 746 doctors in general practice at that time, 513 wrote no prescriptions for either preparation and 243 doctors wrote between 1 and 4 prescriptions in the month. There were a few doctors, however, who were much heavier prescribers of chloramphenicol. Indeed one quarter of all the chloramphenicol prescribed in the whole province was prescribed by 10 doctors. A further study was made in February 1964: this showed that the pattern of prescribing remained the same and in most instances the high prescriber of 1962 was still the high prescriber in 1964.

Because of the anxiety that amphetamines and anti-obesity remedies were being misused in the community (Connell, 1958, Wade and Gibson, 1965) the prescribing of

11 preparations containing amphetamine and phenmetrazine was investigated (Hood and Wade, 1968) over a 3 month period April–June, 1966. In this study a unit of amphetamine was defined as the "equivalent" of 5 mg. of amphetamine. It was found that 11,400 prescriptions were written in the period for almost a million units of amphetamine. There were, however, great differences between the 444 practices (Table 8.1). There were 56 practices (12 per cent. of all practices) in which no amphetamines were prescribed. In 370 practices (85 per cent. of all practices) between 1–2,999 units per 1,000 patients per 3 months were prescribed. There were 18 practices (4 per cent. of all practices) in which between 3,000–10,000 units per 1,000 patients per 3 months were prescribed. These 4 per cent. of the practices were responsible for 20 per cent. of the total prescribing of amphetamines within the province.

These studies and others (Wade and Hood, 1972; Wade, Hood and Haddon, 1973) have shown not only that there

TABLE 8.1

PRESCRIBING OF AMPHETAMINES APRIL–JUNE 1966

Units prescribed /1,000 list patients	Practices prescribing amphetamines		Units of amphetamine prescribed	
	No.	%	No.	%
0	56	12·6		
1–999	293	66·1	302,794	33
1000–1999	48	10·8	210,175	23
2000–2999	28	6·3	226,066	24
3000–3999	6	1·4	53,594	6·0
4000–4999	7	1·6	78,675	8·0
5000–5999	3	0·7	26,671	3·0
6000–6999	1	0·2	20,089	2·0
7000–7999	—	—	—	—
8000–8999	1	0·2	9,745	1·0
Total	433	100%	927,809	100%

are great differences in the use of a drug in different practices but that these differences persist. Although it is sensible for a doctor to prescribe a preparation with which he is familiar, it is disturbing how long a lag exists after the recognition of a serious adverse reaction to a drug before its use is appropriately modified. It is clear that much more thought is needed on the best way to disseminate new information about drugs already in use. Perhaps the torrent of drug promotional literature is a factor in diverting the attention of doctors from more important information about specific drugs, information which they require if their patients are to be treated as effectively and safely as possible.

Changes of prescribing with time

Concern about the misuse and the hazards of certain drugs led to studies in Northern Ireland which have thrown interesting light on the way in which the pattern of prescribing may change with time.

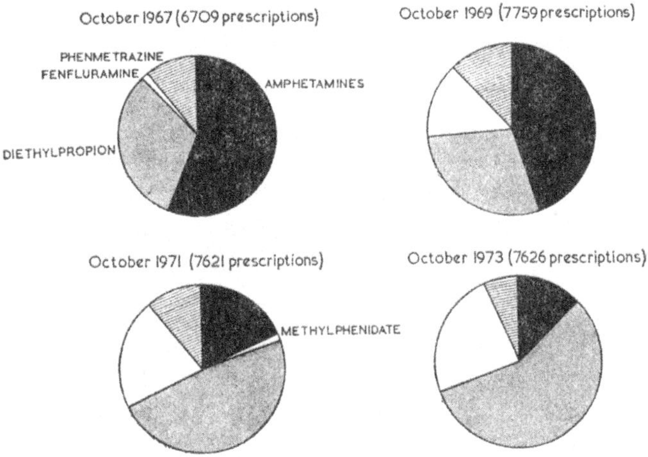

Fig. 8.1. The prescribing of amphetamines and appetite suppressants in Northern Ireland 1967–73. The decrease in the use of amphetamines has been accompanied by increasing use of other appetite suppressant drugs.

Amphetamines. The use of these drugs was kept under monthly review from 1966 to 1971. Figure 8.1 shows the great decrease in the use of these drugs over that period of time. Although this is encouraging, a previous survey by Moorhead (1968) showed that the use of amphetamines by hospital doctors had almost ceased as early as 1963. Despite this between 1963 and 1966 there was a considerable increase in the use of amphetamines in general practice. This is further evidence of the slowness with which new information about the adverse reactions of drugs permeates our profession.

Pressurised aerosols. Another interesting study was made of the use of pressurised aerosols of sympathetico-mimetic drugs. These were first marketed as remedies for bronchospasm in 1959. They were effective and convenient and their use increased rapidly. In 1968 Speizer, Doll and Heaf showed that over the time that the use of these aerosols was increasing, there was an increase in deaths from asthma. This was especially marked in young patients age 10–14 and in many instances the circumstances of death suggested the patient had taken a gross overdose of the aerosol. In June 1967 steps were taken by the Committee on Safety of Drugs to warn doctors of this hazard, warnings against excess use of the aerosol were printed on the containers and the sale of aerosols was limited to prescription. There was a sharp decrease in the death rate following these steps.

A study of the prescribing of the aerosols was made during this period in Northern Ireland (Wade, 1972). In October 1967 (Fig. 8.2), 4,024 prescriptions were written for bronchodilator aerosols, mainly for *PIB* (isoprenaline) *Medihaler Iso Forte* (isoprenaline), and *Medihaler Epi* (adrenaline). A few prescriptions were written for *PIB Forte*. Between 1966 and 1971 the number of different preparations available increased and in October 1973 there were 9,544 prescriptions for 15 preparations. More than half of these were for the newly introduced drugs Orciprenaline, *Alupent*, and salbutamol, *Ventolin*, which were believed to be free of the cardiac stimulant action of isoprenaline and adrenaline, or for sodium chromoglycate, *Intal*, which is not a sympathomimetic drug and acts by interfering with the release of histamine-like substances when allergic reactions occur. The number of prescriptions for aerosols containing isoprenaline or adrenaline did not change as much as might be expected.

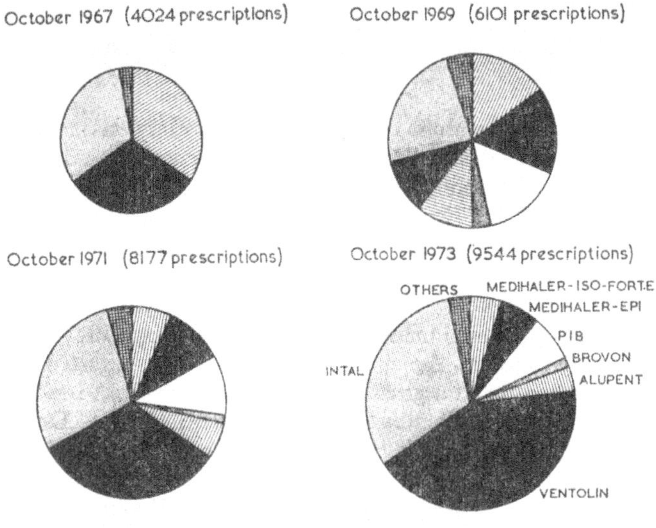

Fig. 8.2. The prescribing of bronchodilator aerosols in Northern Ireland 1967–73.

Hypnotic drugs. A study of the prescribing of hypnotic drugs (Wade and Hood, 1971) from 1966 to 1971 was interesting because in 1965 two new hypnotic preparations were marketed for the first time: *Mandrax*, a preparation containing methaqualone and diphenhydramine, and *Mogadon*, a proprietary preparation of nitrazepam.

The prescribing of *Mandrax* rose rapidly from April 1966, till 1969: its use then declined a little and it was overtaken by *Mogadon*. Fig. 8.3 shows that the prescribing of hypnotic drugs rose from 33,000 prescriptions in October 1966 to 41,000 prescriptions in October 1970.

There was a fourfold increase in the amount of *Mandrax* from 345,000 tablets in 1966 to 1,380,000 tablets in 1969. It was due to more doctors prescribing the preparation, larger numbers of tablets being ordered on each prescription

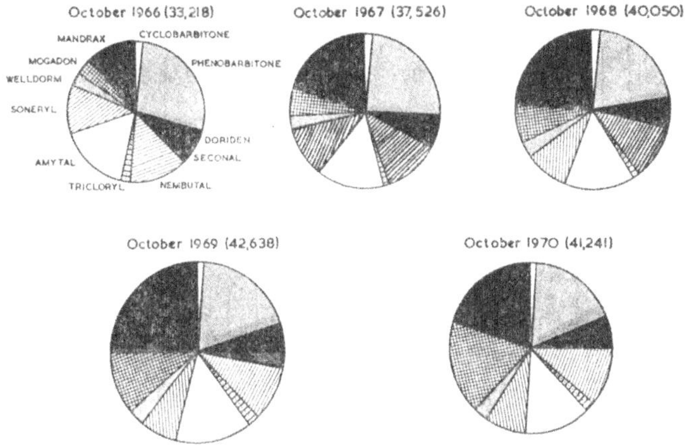

Fig. 8.3. The prescribing of hypnotic drugs in Northern Ireland 1966–1970.

and an increased frequency of prescribing. In July 1966 there were 76 practices (17 per cent. of all practices) in which no *Mandrax* was prescribed and 26 practices (6 per cent. of the total) where it was prescribed at a rate of more than 800 tablets per 1,000 patients. By 1969 only 12 practices (3 per cent.) prescribed no *Mandrax* and 202 (45 per cent.) prescribed more than 800 tablets per 1,000 patients (Fig. 8.4).

The factors which influence the rise and fall in prescribing of a preparation deserve further study. Perhaps the increase in the prescribing of a new preparation is due to the dissatisfaction of doctors and of patients with the drugs already on the market. Possibly a similar motive and the wish to use something new accounts for the subsequent fall in the volume of prescribing of the new drug when some newer preparation becomes available. These cycles of popularity of different drugs are probably an expression of an expectation of the effectiveness of drugs which can never be achieved.

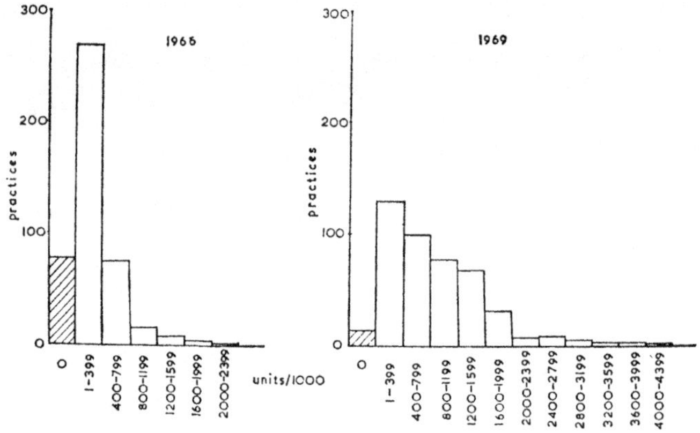

Fig. 8.4. The prescribing of *Mandrax* by practices in Northern Ireland in 1966 and 1969.

It is also important to determine the nature of the information which the individual doctor regards as adequate to justify his use of a new drug or preparation. It seems likely that some doctors are prone to be new drug users. Whether this is because they are easily persuaded by advertisements or whether they are more critical than the rest of us of the adequacy of the drugs previously available is not known.

Geographical differences in prescribing

It has for many years been known that the overall prescribing of drugs varies from area to area in Great Britain, being highest per head of the population in rural areas of Wales, Scotland and Northern Ireland and lowest in the

Midlands (Fig. 8.5). Studies of prescribing in Northern Ireland have shown that there are also great differences in the prescribing of a drug or a group of drugs within quite small regions. Wade, Hadden and Hood (1973) studied the prescribing of antidiabetic drugs over a three month period, April, May and June, 1966. In order to facilitate comparison

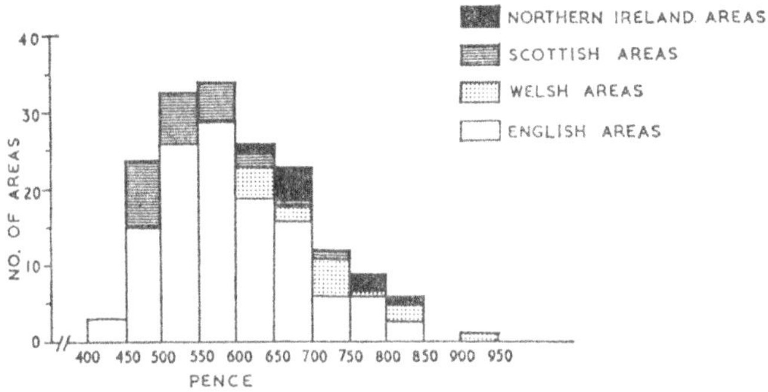

Fig. 8.5. Average total cost per person of prescribed drugs in 1964. England, 123 areas: Wales, 16 areas: Scotland, 25 areas: Northern Ireland, 8 areas.

of the quantities of the different preparations prescribed per 1,000 persons of the population an "equivalent dose" of each preparation was defined (Table 8.2). It was found that during this three month period 3,400 prescriptions for antidiabetic drugs were written a month, 40 per cent. for insulin and 60 per cent. for oral hypoglycaemic drugs. The prescribing of insulin was remarkably constant over the whole province. An average of 3 equivalent doses of insulin, 120 units of insulin, were prescribed per 1,000 patients on doctors lists per day. Prescribing in each of the 6 counties was fairly close to the average. The greatest deviations were in Counties Antrim and Londonderry where it was 28 per cent. and 20 per cent. above the average and the City of Belfast where it was 26 per cent. below the average (Table 8.3).

TABLE 8.2

ANTIDIABETIC PREPARATIONS INCLUDED IN SURVEY AND THEIR CONVERSION TO "EQUIVALENT DOSES" OF APPROXIMATELY ONE DAY'S REQUIREMENTS

Preparation	One "Equivalent Dose"
Insulin	40 units
Metformin (Glucophage)	2 g.
Phenformin (Dibotin, DBI)	50 mg.
Tolbutamide (Rastinon, Orinase)	1 g.
Chlorpropamide (Diabinese)	250 mg.

For oral hypoglycaemic drugs an average of 2,055 prescriptions were written each month, 54 per cent. of them for chlorpropamide, 38 per cent. for tolbutamide and 11 per cent. for metformin. This is an average of 2·7 equivalent doses of the oral hypoglycaemic drugs per 1,000 of the population per day. Figure 8.6 is a map which shows that prescribing of these drugs per head of the population tends to be higher in the east than the west of the province. In Counties Down and Armagh prescribing of these drugs was 36 per cent. and 30 per cent. respectively above the average and in Co. Fermanagh it was 48 per cent. below the average. These differences from the average were much greater for oral hypoglycaemic drugs than had been found for insulin and an attempt to investigate their cause was made.

Londonderry and Newry were chosen for further investigation. In both cities the prescribing of insulin per 1,000 persons on doctors' lists was similar to the provincial mean. But Londonderry was a city in which the use of the oral hypoglycaemics was much lower than the provincial average and Newry was a city in which the use was much higher than the average. Table 8.4 shows that 132 equivalent doses of oral hypoglycaemic drugs/1,000 persons/3 months were prescribed in Londonderry. In Newry 411 equivalent doses/1,000 persons/3 months were prescribed. Further investigation revealed that in each town the same proportion of the

TABLE 8.3

DISTRIBUTION OF PRESCRIBING OF INSULIN AND ORAL HYPOGLYCAEMICS AND OF POPULATION IN COUNTIES OF NORTHERN IRELAND DURING A THREE-MONTH PERIOD IN 1966

	Population*		Insulin		Tablets	
	Number	Percent	'Equivalent' Doses	'Equivalent Doses '/1,000 per Day	'Equivalent Doses'	'Equivalent Doses'/1,000 per Day
Belfast	513,958	36%	102,605	2·2	126,667	2·7
Co. Antrim	238,849	17%	82,065	3·8	57,613	2·7
Co. Armagh	107,663	7%	31,035	3·2	34,646	3·6
Co. Down	223,870	16%	64,762	3·2	74,657	3·7
Co. Fermanagh	38,397	3%	9,775	2·8	4,859	1·4
Co. Londonderry	168,566	12%	54,710	3·6	29,610	1·9
Co. Tyrone	135,847	9%	39,315	3·2	21,820	1·8
Whole Province	1,427,150	100%	384,267	3·0	349,872	2·7

* Northern Ireland Registrar General (1968)

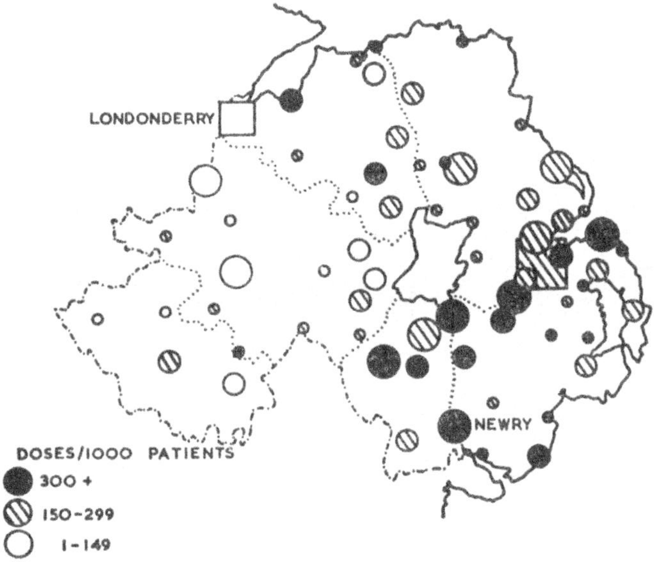

Fig. 8.6. Geographical distribution of prescribing of oral hypoglycaemic drugs in Northern Ireland April–June 1966. The Cities of Belfast and Londonderry are represented by squares and the remaining towns by circles whose size is proportional to the population.

TABLE 8.4

DETAILS OF DIABETIC PATIENTS IN LONDONDERRY AND NEWRY OBTAINED FROM PRESCRIPTION SCRIPTS FOR A THREE-MONTH PERIOD IN 1966

	Londonderry	Newry
Total number of persons on doctor's lists	75,707	30,599
"Equivalent Doses" of oral hypoglycaemics prescribed/1,000 population	132	411
Patients whose prescriptions for oral hypoglycaemics were located	M 34 F 67 } 101	M 12 F 25 } 37
Patients receiving hypoglycaemic therapy/1,000 population	1·33	1·21
Average age (years)	62	63

total population were receiving oral antidiabetic drugs. The greater use of the drugs in Newry was because patients there received much higher daily doses of hypoglycaemic drugs than did patients in Londonderry. The most likely cause for this was that in Londonderry the diabetic physician was able to call on the services of a trained dietician, but in Newry there was no dietician. It seems probable that in Derry control of the blood sugar was being achieved by smaller doses of these oral hypoglycaemic drugs than in Newry because there was greater supervision of the patients' diets.

A number of other studies in Northern Ireland of the use of thyroid and thyroxine, anti-thyroid drugs, antihypertensive drugs and vitamin B_{12} confirmed that great variations in the use of drugs occurred in different areas of the province. It is as though all around us there are therapeutic experiments being conducted of which we have not been aware.

International differences in prescribing

One of the first international studies of drug use was commissioned by the World Health Organisation and carried out by Engels and Siderius (1969). They found that the pattern of prescribing of antibiotics differed greatly in the six European countries they visited. In most countries chloramphenicol was not much used, but in Western Germany it represented 25 per cent. of all antibiotics used (Table 8.5).

In 1971 a WHO Working Party on Drug Consumption met in Oslo. A study was planned to determine whether the differences in prescribing found in different areas in Northern Ireland by Wade and Hood (1972) still existed and whether similar differences occurred in Norway and Sweden. Three groups of drugs were examined.

(A) Drugs essential for the treatment of defined diseases such as insulin and Vitamin B_{12}.

(B) Drugs essential for the management of serious disease but also used in situations where there is doubt about

TABLE 8.5

PERCENTAGE OF SALES OF ANTIBIOTICS IN EUROPE 1966–67

	France	U.K.	Fed. Rep. G.	Belgium	Sweden	Netherlands
Penicillins	20	35	45	11	55	30
Ampicillins	1	15	5	13	15	30
Tetracyclines	40	35	20	20	25	30
Macrolides	8	5	1	30	2	2
Combined tetracyclines and macrolides	8	2	1	15	0	1
Chloramphenicol	5	1	25	1	1	1
Others	18	7	3	10	2	6

(Engels and Siderius 1968)

their value such as antihypertensive drugs, the oral hypoglycaemics, anticoagulants and antidepressants.

(C) Drugs used for symptoms which are not life threatening and which may be meeting the expectations of patients more than filling a medical need. Included here were minor sedatives, hypnotics and tranquillisers.

The data for this survey are still being analysed but some of the preliminary results are available in the three groups.

(A) **Insulin.** The use of insulin (Table 8.6) in Norway and Northern Ireland is approximately the same 3·58 and 3·70 doses/1,000 persons/day. But in Sweden consumption is twice as high 6·93 doses/1,000/persons/day. Use in the seven different areas in Northern Ireland and in eight areas of Sweden was remarkably even, but in Norway the consumption in the Northern areas (26–29) tended to be less than in the rest of the country.

Vitamin B_{12}. The situation of Vitamin B_{12} was very different (Table 8.6). In Sweden on 0·77 daily doses/ 1,000 persons/day were used. Norway used a little more

TABLE 8.6

PRESCRIBING DRUGS IN NORWAY, SWEDEN AND NORTHERN IRELAND
(Daily doses/1000 persons in community/day)

	NORWAY				SWEDEN				NORTHERN IRELAND		
	Daily doses/1,000/day				Daily doses/1,000/day				Daily doses/1,000/day		
Area	Insulin	Oral Hypo	Vit.B_{12}	Area	Insulin	Oral Hypo	Vit.B_{12}	Area	Insulin	Oral Hypo	Vit.B_{12}
11	4·71	9·55	1·38	1	6·57	12·60	1·00	1	3·17	3·55	4·16
12	3·16	6·15	0·63	2	7·17	18·40	·77	2	4·29	4·70	3·83
13	4·25	12·77	1·87	3	8·00	19·53	·77	3	3·17	5·44	8·09
14	3·59	8·98	1·03	4	6·70	11·13	·77	4	4·29	4·85	4·75
15	3·52	5·45	0·72	5	6·20	14·77	·67	5	3·53	3·76	5·18
16	4·11	8·33	2·52	6	7·00	17·13	1·00	6	3·60	3·58	2·71
17	3·49	4·89	1·17	7	6·90	16·87	·43	7	3·76	3·66	3·04
18	4·26	6·75	2·12	J	6·90	18·80	1·43				
19	4·18	10.11	1.11								
21	3·50	5.66	1·32								
22	3·55	4·85	·88								
23	3·01	6·55	·58								
24	2·05	6·15	·61								
25	3·90	5·72	·64								
26	4·73	8·54	·74								
27	2·83	6·74	·57								
28	2·53	7·92	·45								
29	1·42	5·26	·39								
MEAN	3·58	7·16	1·02		6·93	15·17	0·77		3·70	4·14	4·26

1·02 daily doses/1,000 persons/day. In Northern Ireland consumption was six times greater than in Sweden, 4·26 daily doses/1,000 persons/day (Fig. 8.7). The variation within each country is also great, with areas where the use is as small as 40 per cent. below the average and as large as 70 per cent. above the average in each country. In Northern Ireland the use of Vitamin B_{12} was highest in the more remote rural areas 3 and 5.

The use of the oral antidiabetic drugs is shown diagramatically in Fig. 8.8. Consumption is higher in Sweden, 15·27 daily.doses/1,000 persons/day than in Norway, 7·16 daily doses/1,000 persons/ day, and in Northern Ireland consumption is only 4·33 daily doses/1,000 persons/day (Table 8.6). In each country there are great variations in the choice of biguanides and sulphonylureas.

B The consumption of potent oral hypotensive drugs was found to be highest in Sweden 9·13 daily doses/1,000 persons/day. In Northern Ireland it was 7·00 daily doses/1,000 persons/day and in Norway it was 4·36 daily doses/1,000 persons/day—almost half the Swedish use. It was unexpectedly found that the use of these drugs was less in urban areas of Northern Ireland and Sweden than in rural areas. In Norway where the over all use is much lower the highest consumption was in Oslo.

Methyldopa was the most popular drug in all three countries at the time of the survey. The blocking agents bethanidine and guanethidine were the next most popular drugs in Norway and Northern Ireland, but in Sweden hydrallazine was used twice as often as the blocking agents. At the time of the study debrisoquine was in use only in Northern Ireland and clonidine was being used only in Norway and Sweden.

C The use of these drugs has increased greatly in the last few years and amongst them are included the most frequently prescribed individual drugs in each country. In Norway consumption was 35·2 doses/1,000 persons/

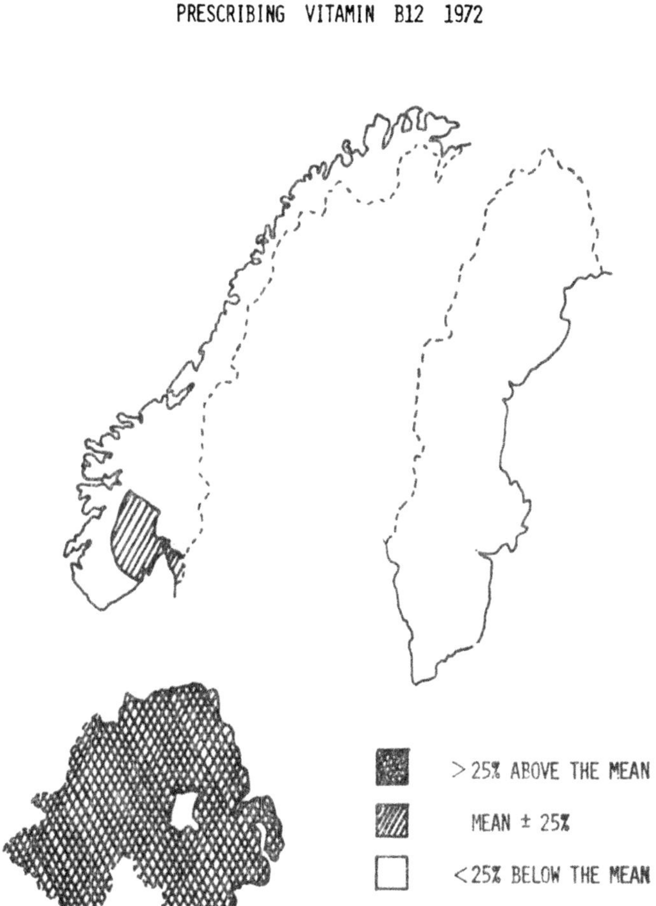

Fig. 8.7. The prescribing of vitamin B_{12} preparations in areas of Norway, Sweden and Northern Ireland in 1972.

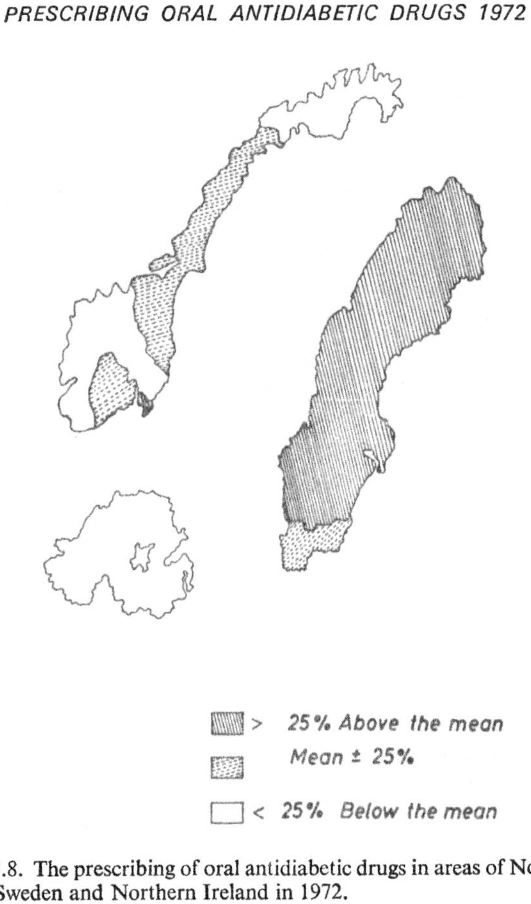

Fig. 8.8. The prescribing of oral antidiabetic drugs in areas of Norway, Sweden and Northern Ireland in 1972.

day, in Northern Ireland it was 32·6 daily doses/1,000 persons/day. Figures for Sweden are not yet available except for one County. Here it was 26·3 daily doses/1,000 persons/day. In both Norway and Northern Ireland the use of these drugs was much higher in urban areas than in rural areas. Consumption in Norway seems to have levelled off in the last year or so, but in Northern Ireland it is still rising.

This survey has shown as was expected that in Norway and Sweden there are geographical variations in drug use similar to those Wade and Hood found in Northern Ireland. What was not expected was that the differences in the use of some drugs between countries were much greater than the differences within them.

Conclusion

Monitoring adverse reactions to drugs presents many problems that are yet to be solved. Doctors need clear, concise, unbiased information about drugs, including information about the nature and frequency of any serious adverse reactions. Knowledge about this, about the use of drugs and about their value when they are used in a modern community is too often not available. The methods by which this knowledge may be obtained and disseminated have not yet been developed and the will to develop them is not yet apparent.

The major difficulty is that there are a number of conflicting beliefs and anxieties held by society of which any worker in clinical pharmacology soon becomes aware.

Many people have an expectation of remedies which exceeds what is possible. This is especially true of patients and their relatives in the discomfort, fear and sorrow of serious illness. But it is true also of many doctors. It is disturbing how many doctors will continue to believe, some passionately, in the merits of medication in the absence of any convincing proof of merit. It is disturbing too that so often when a new drug is introduced it is acclaimed with an enthusiasm which past experience shows is unjustifiable.

Perhaps it is because there is a large element of faith behind our acceptance of the effectiveness of contemporary therapy that doctors unconsciously, sometimes consciously, resent adverse reactions to drugs. If it is disturbing to learn that the therapy we give to our patients to make them better is of no value, it is even more disturbing to learn, that it is harming them.

There are others in society who underrate the benefits of drug therapy. They fear adverse reactions, exaggerate their importance, see all drugs as potential heirs to thalidomide, resent the cavalier behaviour of doctors who thoughtlessly prescribe medicaments instead of spending time and trouble with anxious, worried or dis-eased patients, suspect the drug industry of promulgating the use of meretricious preparations and sometimes hanker for a past in which simple virtues are imagined to have reigned supreme and stability and conformity to have been unchallenged by change. They wish that there were no problems of drug abuse, no controversy about the use of contraceptives by the unmarried, no anxieties that psychotropic drugs were sapping the moral fibre of the masses and no concern lest the present use of drugs should hazard the genetic health of future generations.

It is extremely important that these problems are seen in proper perspective. Modern drugs have changed the face of medicine during the last three decades and doctors would not like to practice medicine without them. The good drugs have done outweighs the evil. The adverse reactions to drugs must be seen in the perspective of the other hazards of modern life, the aeroplane, the automobile, the use of tobacco and the consumption of alcohol. Emotional reactions do not help us to solve the difficult problems of monitoring adverse reactions to drugs.

CHAPTER IX

DRUG REGULATORY BODIES AND THEIR PROBLEMS

The thalidomide catastrophe marked the beginning of a period of increasing public concern about the dangers of drugs, food additives and pesticides. In a number of countries new laws were passed or existing legislation was modified to ensure that there was supervision of drugs put on the market. Evidence was required that they were effective for the purposes the manufacturer claimed, that in the context of the diseases for which they were to be used they were safe and that their specifications and purity were acceptable. Looking at the work of the drug regulatory bodies which exist at present, it is possible to define an underlying philosophy.

The Philosophy of Drug Regulatory Bodies

All drug regulatory bodies accept that it is their duty to:

1. *Examine toxicity data.* The pharmacological and toxicological work carried out by the manufacturer is assessed to confirm that adequate toxicity tests have been done to justify the administration of the drug to patients for clinical trial and that there is sufficient evidence of likely therapeutic value.

Usually a clinical trials certificate is issued. Often the protocol of these trials has to be approved, the centres at which they are to be conducted may be named and the number of trials and their duration limited.

2. *Assess Clinical Trials.* The results of clinical trials, and sometimes of further long term animal toxicity tests which have been carried out, are examined to determine whether the drug may be marketed.

3. *Issue licences.* In many countries a licence is needed by the manufacturer for each preparation which he markets. Usually the uses for which the drug is to be promoted and the nature of any warnings thought to be necessary are agreed with the manufacturer before a licence is issued.

4. *Supervise specifications and quality.* The pharmaceutical formulation of a preparation is examined to ensure its purity and stability. Details of the tolerances allowed in manufacturing and evidence of the biological availability of the active ingredient may be demanded. The premises at which production of the drug takes place may be examined regularly by inspectors of the licensing authority and random samples of the marketed drug may be taken for analyses.

5. *Monitor adverse reactions.* The establishment of a system which allows the early identification of unforeseen adverse reactions after the drug has been marketed is usually accepted as best done by the national drug regulatory body.

In some countries it is believed that the drug regulatory body should examine the efficacy of a preparation in relation to the other remedies available and should give advice to doctors about their choice of drugs.

Features of Some National Drug Regulatory Bodies

Britain. The first Pure Food and Drugs Act was passed in Britain in 1868. It was followed by a series of Poisons Laws, Dangerous Drugs Acts and Therapeutic Substances Acts. None was suitable to ensure that adequate tests were done to show before marketing that a new drug was safe and after the thalidomide catastrophe the Minister of Health appointed a Committee on Safety of Drugs. Its Chairman was Sir Derrick Dunlop and its members independent experts mainly from Universities and Medical Schools: none were government employees, none worked for the Pharmaceutical Industry and they gave their services without remuneration. The Dunlop Committee held its first meeting on 6th June, 1963. The Committee had no statutory powers but it sought and obtained a voluntary agreement from all pharmaceutical firms in the United Kingdom that no new drug or pharmaceutical preparation would be marketed without its permission. That agreement was strictly honoured, a tribute to the standing of the Committee's Chairman and its members, to the competence of its officers and the probity of the firms. It always amazed our American visitors that a voluntary system could work so well, but perhaps they did not realise that despite an absence of statutory powers the Committee had powerful teeth.

In 1968 the Medicines Act was passed and the Medicines Commission was subsequently appointed. Fig. 9.1 shows the

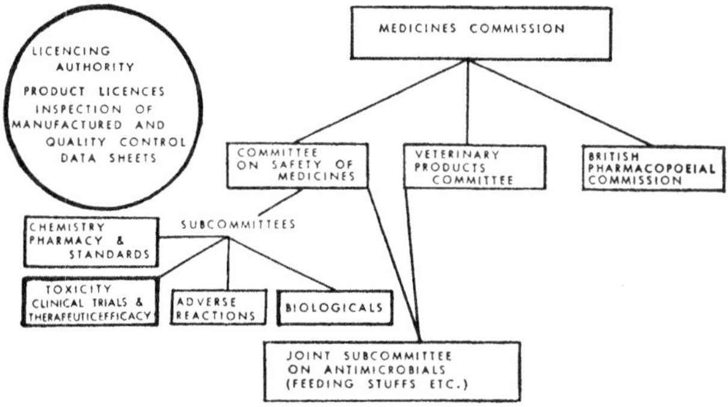

Fig. 9.1

present structure of the British drug regulatory system. The Committee on Safety of Medicines replaced the old Dunlop Committee and there were some changes in procedure. Whereas no manufacturer had been able to appeal against a decision of the Dunlop Committee, he can now appeal from a decision of the Committee on Safety of Medicines to the Medicines Commission. No member of the Medicines Commission may sit on the Committee on Safety of Medicines because he may have to sit in judgement on an appeal. Under the new Act a manufacturer has to obtain a licence for every product he markets. This licence is issued by the Department of Health and Social Security on the advice of the Committee on Safety of Medicines.

The Committee on Safety of Medicines issues guidelines to manufacturers indicating the nature of the evidence that is required before a new drug may be used in clinical trials in patients or may be marketed: data obtained abroad, if of adequate scientific standard, is acceptable to the Committee.

The Dunlop Committee and its successor have always felt that the choice of drug is best left to the doctor looking after the individual patient. This choice is a matter of professional judgement and should be the result of opinion derived from medical and scientific discussion within the profession.

This is a sensible attitude. It is never possible when a drug or preparation is first marketed to predict the place it will take in the medical armamentarium. The use and popularity of a drug may wax or wane, as experience in its use increases, as new concepts of disease develop or as other new drugs are introduced. Thus in the mid 1950's anticoagulant therapy was thought to be important both in the immediate treatment of myocardial infarcation and in prophylactic long term use to prevent recurrences. Experience and the results of well planned controlled therapeutic trials have shown these views to be wrong and anticoagulant therapy is not widely used for myocardial infarcation now in Britain although it still is in some other countries.

Nor is it felt to be the business of the Medicines Commission to dictate to doctors how they should use drugs. This is a matter of professional training and professional competence. It is, however, the concern of the Commission that unbiased information about drugs should be readily available to doctors. Fortunately besides good weekly journals such as the *Lancet* and the *British Medical Journal*, there are publications which deal especially with drugs. *The British National Formulary* is prepared by a Joint Formulary Committee of the British Medical Association and the

Pharmaceutical Society of Great Britain. *Prescribers Journal* is published by the Department of Health but it is managed by an independent editorial board and it carries signed articles by men whose professional standing is itself a warranty of the independence of their views and *The Drugs and Therapeutics Bulletin* is published by the Consumers Association. Under the Medicines Act a drug firm must send to all doctors a "data sheet" about each drug that it markets. The very full and unbiased information included in these data sheets has to be approved by the Licensing Authority. Recently under the aegis of the Association of the British Pharmaceutical Industry a Compendium of the data sheets issued by a number of its member companies has been published and this new and authoritative publication is a most useful source of information.

United States of America. America has the biggest pharmaceutical industry in the world and the Bureau of Drugs of the Food and Drugs Administration (FDA) has a duty placed on it by Congress to ensure that marketed drugs are safe. Manufacturers have to file details of proposed clinical studies of an investigational new drug, IND, but the major hurdle is to get clearance from the FDA of the new drug application, NDA, to allow marketing. There has been serious criticism of the FDA from the pharmaceutical industry and the medical profession that it is both slow and inefficient. Until recently most of the assessment and clearance of NDAs was done by the in-house staff which did not have a high scientific standing. Many of the most knowledgeable and competent scientists and medical men were not invited to help the FDA because they were associated however remotely with industry. This was assumed to interfere with their independence of judgement. Indeed it is a legally indictable offence to advise a governmental body if there is any possibility of a "conflict of interest".

It has not been easy for the FDA to recruit to its staff men of acceptable scientific stature. This has been because the FDA has operated in a highly charged political environment.

Ever since the Kevauver hearings in 1959–62 which revealed evidence of dishonest and unethical practices by some drug firms the decisions of the FDA have been subject to scrutiny by congressional committees, journalists, consumer groups and cranks. Politicians have found it possible to gain publicity by fanning public anxiety with claims that the FDA was allowing the pharmaceutical industry to market drugs which had been inadequately tested. It is not surprising that officers in the FDA became reluctant to make decisions which might lead to criticism and tended to procrastinate. Within the FDA there was a firm belief that there could be no glory in approval and it was not easy to forget that Dr. Kelsey, who held up the marketing of thalidomide for reasons which in retrospect were not at all relevant, was awarded a medal when it was found that the drug was a teratogen. There has been an undue emphasis by the FDA on the ability of premarketing assessment to detect drug toxicity. This perhaps accounts for the enormous size of the submissions that firms send to the FDA: submissions of more than 100 volumes are not uncommon.

When a serious reaction is suspected in a drug that has been passed for marketing, and in the present state of knowledge this cannot be completely avoided, the FDA tends to overreact and its officers have an unhappy reputation of "shooting from the hip".

Another and a serious difficulty is that under the American Constitution if an FDA decision is challenged by a firm, final judgement is obtained by recourse to the courts where there is opposition of legal adversaries; not in the opinion of many, the best arena in which to settle technical and scientific differences.

Australia and Canada. In both these countries the philosophy of the drug regulatory bodies is nearer to the British than the American pattern. The Australian Drug Evaluation Committee is a group of medical scientists of high standing drawn from Universities and professional bodies and they advise the Department of Health which is the licensing body but which has a skilled if small professional secretariate. Outside experts are called on readily. There are subcommittees of the Drug Evaluation Committee concerned with adverse reactions of drugs, congenital abnormalities and vaccines. A separate body, the Pharmaceutical Benefits Committee, makes decisions as to the relative efficacy of marketed drugs in the course of deciding for the Department of Health which drugs should be placed on the drug tariff and may be prescribed by doctors at no cost to their patients.

In Canada the Food and Drugs Directorate has established its own laboratory at Ottawa and carries out its own studies on the biological availability of drugs in the formulations marketed by different firms. It also publishes an excellent Bulletin, in English and French, with comments about contemporary drug problems and data sheets of newly marketed drugs.

Germany, Switzerland and Japan. The Federal Republic of Germany is the second largest pharmaceutical producer in the world. The pharmaceutical industry is strong and efficient and preclinical toxicological work is done by them most efficiently. Clinical pharmacology is, however, almost non-existent, clinical trials are not a dominant part of the medical scene and the drug regulatory system has been until very recently derisory. Even now there is no requirement that firms have to obtain clearance before clinical trials are carried out and approval before marketing is slow because the Department of Drugs is very small and has an enormous backlog of work (as of Jan. 1974). It does not help that the Department of Drugs is sited in Berlin far away from the centres of industry, and that political considerations make it unlikely that this can be changed.

Switzerland is another giant of drug production but its drug regulatory body is a pygmy. The small Federal Control Office does, however, have excellent relations with industry. As in Germany, firms do not have to have clearance of a new drug before carrying out clinical trials but approval is needed before the new drug is marketed.

Japan already has a substantial drug industry: it is growing rapidly and beginning to challenge the export markets of the world. All pharmaceutical preparations marketed in Japan have to be registered with the Pharmaceutical Affairs Council. One of the difficulties of foreign firms which wish to market drugs in Japan is that the Council requires data to have been obtained in laboratories or hospitals in Japan.

The Problems of Drug Regulatory Bodies

Delay

Drug regulatory bodies have such a heavy burden of work that there are always complaints about the delay they cause to firms wishing to develop and market new drugs (*see* Table 9.1). Complaints have been especially common in the U.S.A. Drugs such as cotrimoxazole (*Septrin* and *Bactrim*), sodium chromoglycate (*Intal*) and salbutamol (*Ventolin*) were marketed for many years in Britain before marketing permission was obtained in the U.S.A. and American physicians have justifiably complained that the FDA in its efforts to ensure the safety of drugs has denied American citizens the drugs they need.

TABLE 9.1

	Certificate required for clinical trial	Average time needed to obtain certificate	Approval for marketing required	Average time needed to obtain approval for marketing
Australia	yes	6-12 months	yes	2-3 years
Germany	no	—	yes	2-3 years
Japan	no	—	yes	1 year
Sweden	yes	2 weeks	yes	2 years
Switzerland	no	—	yes	4 months
United Kingdom	yes	6 months	yes	6 months
United States	yes	1 month	yes	2 years

Information obtained in November 1973.

Some of the delay is the fault of firms who send incomplete or inadequate submissions, some is due to slow communication within very large organisations like the large international drug firms and the bigger of the drug regulatory bodies. It was admitted in 1970 that in the FDA it took two weeks for a document from a firm to pass through the mail room. If a document carried legal weight it was first stamped with the date and time of receipt and the front page bearing the stamp was xeroxed and returned to the firm as an acknowledgement of receipt. The document was then indexed and cross indexed, so that it would be easily retrieved and a copy was deposited in the library files. When this is finished, and it may take two weeks, the letter may still have to be routed through various offices and divisions until it reaches the man it is addressed to. This is the routine of most American Government Offices and it is at least encouraging that the FDA officers are aware of the problem and as anxious as anyone to deal with it.

Inhibition of innovation

It has been claimed, mainly in the U.S.A. but in other countries as well including Britain, that the activities of the drug regulatory bodies have impaired if not stifled the innovation and development of new drugs. The Vice-president of one American firm said "many firms have precious little research management talent and these people have been diverted to dealing with the FDA problem and they are not managing research back in the shop" (Gilgore, 1970). The Director of Research of Ciba has stated that whereas in the early 1960's it took two years from the discovery of guanethidine (Ismelin) to its marketing, in 1970 it would now take between six and seven years (de Stevens, 1970).

But these complaints of "regulatory overkill" may be exaggerated. There are others who believe that drug innovation in the late 1960's slowed down because there was a drying up of the fundamental knowledge which must precede innovation and an increasing preoccupation by industry with "me-tooism", the non-creative duplication of the existing products made by other manufacturers.

It will probably not be fair for many years to make

judgement as to whether innovation has been inhibited but there is no doubt that the establishment of drug regulatory bodies has led in the last ten years to a great improvement in the quality and quantity of toxicological and pharmacological work done before a new drug is marketed: indeed there is real anxiety that some of the work now being demanded adds little to the safety of the drug and that the pharmaceutical industry may be unnecessarily burdened with many of the tests which are routinely demanded.

The glare of publicity

On 20th May, 1970 when the preliminary results of the University Group Diabetic Program first became available, Morton Mintz, columnist of the Washington Post fired off one of those American shots which are heard around the world. He wrote "a massive study of patients with mild diabetes indicates that if they take the most popular anti-diabetic pills (tolbutamide) for more than three years they are more likely to die prematurely than if they take insulin or no medication at all. The study . . . suggests . . . that at least 8,000 users of the drug die prematurely every year in the United States alone".

The next day, 21st May, the FDA issued a warning about the hazards of all sulphonylurea drugs. When this hasty statement was later criticised because it was made before there had been adequate discussion of the results by the medical and scientific community, Dr. Jennings, an Associate Commissioner of the FDA, said "We could not afford that luxury (the delay) when a lay newspaper declared that 8,000 more patients would die this year as a result of taking the drug".

This sorry story raises many issues. The investigators intended to present their data at a scientific meeting of the American Diabetic Association and then to publish them in a scientific journal for discussion in an appropriate scientific and medical forum. Instead the issue was discussed in the ill-informed and inappropriate public forum of the TV and press. It was discussed in an emotional and unbalanced fashion. The officers of the FDA in the glare of publicity, acccepted at face value the comment of a lay journalist that 8,000 users of the drug would die prematurely in the next year, a comment which was unjustified on the data available—indeed after four years of further study there is still argument as to the interpretation of the data.

In Britain similar unfortunate premature publicity occurred when the data collected about adverse reactions to the oral contraceptive pills showed that the small incidence of thromboembolism was related to the oestrogen content of the preparations. When the analysis of these results was presented to the Adverse Reactions Sub-Committee on Thursday, 23rd October 1969, it was recommended that the data should be prepared for publication in one of the medical journals and that a letter outlining the findings should be sent to every doctor. The Committee on Safety of Drugs accepted these recommendations at its next meeting on 27th November and by that time a draft of the statement to be sent to doctors was available and was modified in the light of suggestions of the members.

Through no fault of the Committee there was delay. The statement had to be printed by Her Majesty's Stationery Office and envelopes had to be addressed to all doctors, an exercise never previously carried out by the Department of Health. This was done by the second weekend in December and the Post Office confirmed that if posted by Saturday, 13th December the statement would reach all doctors, except a few in the Highlands, by the morning of Monday, 15th December.

Because the manufacturers would need to know of the prescribing changes that were going to be recommended to doctors a meeting of the medical advisers of firms that manufactured the oral contraceptives was called. It was held on the afternoon of Wednesday, 10th December, and those present were asked to consider the information as confidential until Monday, 15th December when all doctors would have received information about the findings. Within a few hours of the end of that meeting Chapman Pincher of the Daily Express rang one of the officers of the Committee on Safety of Drugs, gave an accurate account of the statement, asked if his information was correct and had it printed on the front page of the Daily Express the next morning, Thursday, 11th December under the headline "Safer birth pill. Doctors find way". Because of the demand for information by other journalists and newsmen the Department of Health and Social Security brought forward to that afternoon a press conference arranged for Monday, 15th December.

Thus the public heard of the new information about oral contraceptives from the media, and many newspapers presented it in a more dramatic and less satisfactory form than did Chapman Pincher's article. It created quite extraordinary and unnecessary public anxiety so that on Friday, 13th, and Saturday, 14th December, thousands of women descended on their family doctors who had not yet received the official statement and indeed due to miscalculation by the Post Office who had forgotten the build up of Christmas mail, were not to receive it in many instances until 18th or 19th December.

So it was that a statement about oral contraceptive preparations made with the intention of marginally improving the safety of the use of such preparations was interpreted by many of our public as demonstrating that some of the preparations on the market were highly dangerous. The doctors who could have assuaged their fears had not been informed and were infuriated by what appeared to them as the incompetence and hamhandedness of the Committee on Safety of Drugs.

Emotion and the glare of publicity impair judgement and increase the likelihood of erroneous decisions. There is no doubt that if the officers of a public body are aware of this they can often take steps to avoid putting themselves in a position in which they have to make decisions in a difficult and exposed situation. It is in our opinion mandatory to publish the data on which decisions are made at the same time as any statement is made. This is now the policy of the Committee on Safety of Medicines and since its adoption a number of important statements about adverse reactions to drugs have been made without stirring inappropriate and unnecessary public anxiety.

Limitations

Despite the hopes of the public and comforting words of statesmen, the existence of a drug regulatory body will never completely abolish the hazard that accompanies the use of new drugs in human beings. However much work is done in preclinical testing, absolute safety can never be guaranteed and if a serious adverse reaction only occurs infrequently it may well be missed before a new drug is marketed. There will always be argument about how much premarketing testing should be demanded by drug regulatory bodies and it is always going to be difficult to balance the requirements of safety against the need for new medication. Sometimes the need is great especially if existing therapy is unsatisfactory.

After a drug has been marketed all drug regulatory bodies have found that they need the cooperation and support of the medical profession and others to report to them suspected adverse reactions to drugs. No one has yet shown how this cooperation may be increased—at present it is everywhere inadequate.

However competent a drug regulatory body may be it cannot usurp the position of the individual medical practitioner. It cannot dictate to a doctor the remedy he should choose to treat his patient—that is a decision best made by the man familiar with the patient and his complaint. Nor can it prevent the misuse of drugs. A very good drug may be used in inappropriate circumstances. No regulatory body can play any effective part in handling that problem—its correction lies in the quality of man who is selected for training as a medical practitioner and the calibre of training that he receives.

CHAPTER X

THE FUTURE

A decade is a short time but in the years since the thalidomide catastrophe adverse reactions to drugs have become of deep concern to doctors, pharmacologists, the pharmaceutical industry and governmental drug regulatory bodies. It is difficult to assess the effect of these developments on the attitude of the community to drugs, for this remains strangely ambivalent.

On the one hand the public demands medicines with undiminished enthusiasm. Their politicians remain as anxious as ever that the National Health Service should meet this demand although they express concern about costs and make numerous suggestions as to how these may be reduced. Many doctors still prescribe drugs with an intemperance and readiness which suggest that neither rational therapy, the incidence of adverse reactions to drugs nor the cost to the Health Service is much on their mind. Moreover criticism of their prescribing is much resented by many doctors. "The freedom of the doctor to prescribe what his patient needs" is quite rightly defended with vigour as a bulwark of a professional freedom which might be lost if bureaucracy were allowed to intrude. Yet it is a pity that this virtuous sentiment should give dignity to prescribing which is thoughtless and excessive, especially as some money at present spent on pharmaceutical services might be spent to better effect on other parts of the Health Service.

On the other hand many people see adverse reactions to drugs as an ominous threat to the nation's health. They uncritically demand restrictions on the prescribing of drugs by doctors and advocate such exhaustive and long lasting tests on new drugs that the development of new therapy would be impeded.

History teaches us that views which differ so greatly as this attentuate with time. Although it is difficult to predict the future with accuracy there are some developments which seem likely to occur during the next decade.

1. New developments in the assessment of drugs

Before a new drug is marketed for use in man extensive animal toxicity tests, pharmacokinetic studies, investigations of the mode of its action and trials of its effectiveness in comparison with existing therapy are carried out. But to date there has been no critical examination of the cost benefits of such work. How much of the toxicity work currently demanded by the Committee on Safety of Medicines or the Food and Drugs Administration is really necessary? How much is of little value and gives a spurious sense of security to the community? Pharmaceutical firms are reluctant to discuss the compounds which they initially hoped would be useful drugs but which had to be put aside because tests showed that they might be dangerous. Yet if toxicity tests are to be improved this data and much information filed by governmental drug regulatory bodies which is at present confidential, needs to be critically reviewed. This will surely happen: the resulting improvement in tests and the reduction in their number will be of economic advantage to the pharmaceutical industry, and will improve the safety of drugs.

2. Operational research

Studies on the prescribing and use of individual drugs and of the incidence of adverse reactions will be extended. At present Sweden leads the world in this work. Although work on contraception of the very highest quality is being supported by the Medical Research Council under the supervision of Professor Doll and Professor Vessey at Oxford, the Department of Health and Social Security has to date shown little interest in investigations of the effective use of drugs. Little attempt is being made at present in England and Wales to examine and analyse the use of drugs by general practitioners, although they prescribe more than 95 per cent. of all drugs used in the country. However a small number of drug safety officers have been appointed in hospitals and it is intended that in the Health Service there should be appointed physicians with a special interest in clinical pharmacology. Such appointments could play an important role in improving the use and safety of drugs.

3. Improvement in the accessibility of information on drugs

Even when extensive information about a new drug is available it is not always easily accessible to those who will prescribe the drug. It may be published in scientific journals of limited circulation or in a form which can only be understood by the few who are experts in drug metabolism or pharmacokinetics. The recently introduced "data sheets" which under the Medicines Act the manufacturer of every preparation has to make available to doctors will help greatly, especially if the layout of the data sheets is improved and the information included is better standardised.

There will, however, continue to be a need for well balanced and well informed criticism of current drug therapy and comparison of one form of treatment with another. Here again it is difficult to make this information easily accessible to practising doctors. There is such a torrent of drug promotional material and such a plethora of journals including many of doubtful integrity which are sent unsolicited that many doctors become disheartened in their efforts to keep up to date.

Ways in which modern data processing equipment might help the prescriber are being investigated in many centres. Information about drugs can be stored in a computer system in such a way as to facilitate easy reference to information which can be kept complete and up to date. Pharmacy-based computer systems have been developed by which prescriptions can be validated before administration and attempts are also being made to use computers to help the prescriber more directly. In one system currently being developed (Beeley, Bishop, Leach and Walker, 1974) relevant drug information stored in a computer is presented to the doctor as he prescribes a drug. Details about the patient and the drugs he is receiving are also stored in the computer and prescriptions can be checked for errors, contraindications and drug interactions before the prescription is completed. No doubt other systems will be developed, for the amount of information that has to be available if some drugs are to be prescribed with safety may become beyond the range of reasonable memory without the help of computers.

4. Regulatory bodies

The Medicines Commission is of recent birth. It and its predecessor the Committee on Safety of Drugs, the Dunlop Committee, have played an important part in improving the safety of drugs. The Commission will face problems of daunting difficulty as new types of drugs are developed. These may include new contraceptives, drugs which increase fertility, drugs which alter sensation, perhaps enhancing taste or smell, and psychotropic drugs which may alter emotions, increase or decrease motivation or modify a sense of guilt. But the Medicines Commission is mainly concerned with the purity, reliability and safety of the drugs. It is not responsible for the proper and sensible use of drugs by doctors, except in as much as the Commission has a duty to ensure that there is full unbiased information about the drugs available to doctors. The responsibility for the proper use of drugs rests with the prescriber, and ultimately the standard of medical care the public receives depends on the calibre and quality of medical practitioners.

The Medical Acts, the first of which was passed in 1858 and under which the General Medical Council receives its authority have never strangely enough stated that it should be the concern of the Council to promote high standards of professional conduct (Annual Report, 1973). It would seem likely, however, that in the near future the Council will begin to take a more active part in relation to the issue of guidance on questions of professional conduct. This may well include guidance about the prescribing of drugs. Although it is at present widely accepted that only a doctor who has had the appropriate training is entitled to undertake major surgical procedures, it is reasonable to expect that it will one day become more widely accepted that there are certain forms of drug therapy which none but those who have specialised knowledge should prescribe, or which should only be prescribed by a doctor in consultation with an expert. Dollery (1971) has argued convincingly that all who work in the health professions must accept that it is proper that their work should be critically scrutinised by independent professional bodies. He believes that unless there is an "audit of health care" there will not be the constant criticism which will raise standards where they are indifferent towards the best—and this will apply as much to prescribing and the use of drugs as to many other facets of our medical services.

5. Changes in the law

At the time of writing the law concerning the liability of drug manufacturers has been challenged by those who claim compensation from Distillers Co. (Biochemicals) who made and sold thalidomide in Britain. The negotiations on this issue (Report by *Sunday Times*, 1973) have continued for ten years within a legal cocoon and discussion of the issues has been limited by the constraints of contempt of court. This is unfortunate. The community needs to have the position clarified. Important as it is for firms to be liable if they are negligent, it is conceivable if the voices of some prevail that public sympathy for these unfortunate children will find expression in a declaration of a degree of liability that will inhibit the innovation of new and perhaps badly needed drugs. It can be predicted that as soon as this case ceases to be *sub judice*, there will be wide discussion on this problem and there are likely to be changes in the law, and perhaps changes in the rights of the unborn child.

6. Changes in attitudes

Attitudes will continue to change. Both the public and the medical profession are increasingly accepting that no drug can be completely safe, that the use of any drug must be justified and that as few drugs as possible should be prescribed at once. There is also an increasing awareness of the importance of clinical pharmacology. Departments of clinical pharmacology have now been established in a number of medical schools and more will be established. It is increasingly appreciated that men with training in this discipline are needed not only in our medical schools, but in our hospitals, in general practice and certainly in industry. At the time of writing both the Health Service and Universities are faced with financial stringency; it is difficult to maintain what is already established, let alone expand and develop a new discipline. It is well known, however, that financial icebergs eventually melt—and it is reasonable to predict that by the end of a decade, by 1984, clinical pharmacology will be a much more important discipline than at present. Those of us who suffer the present frustrations can say with Horace "Dimidium facti qui coepit habet: sapere aude". The task has been begun but is not finished: have the courage to be wise.

APPENDIX I

ADVERSE REACTIONS TO DRUGS

These lists are arranged according to the classification of drugs used in the British National Formulary. Although most of the important known adverse reactions are included, the lists are not comprehensive. Further information can be found in the list of references at the end of the appendix. Reactions which are produced by a group of drugs are listed under the group name. Examples of specific drugs belonging to the group are given but the lists are not necessarily complete.

ALIMENTARY SYSTEM

Antacids	Calcium salts and absorbable alkalis can produce hypercalcaemia and renal failure —"milk alkali syndrome".
Carbenoxolone	Oedema. Hypertension. Cardiac failure. Hypokalaemia. Muscle weakness.
Antispasmodics	
Atropine Belladona Hyoscine Propantheline Dicyclomine	Dry mouth. Constipation. Urinary retention. Blurred vision — may precipitate glaucoma. Mental confusion.
Laxatives	Excessive use may cause dehydration, hypokalaemia and megacolon (irritant ones only).

Senna	Melanosis coli after prolonged use.
Danthron	Red urine.
Liquid paraffin	Malabsorption of fat-soluable vitamins. Paraffinoma.
Phenolphthalein	Pink urine. Rashes, including fixed eruptions.
Oxyphenisatin	Jaundice.

ANTI-EMETICS

Anti-histamines	
Cyclizine Meclozin Diphenhydramine Promethazine Dimenhydrinate	Drowsiness. Potentiate all sedatives and alcohol. Dry mouth and blurred vision. Skin sensitisation.
Hyoscine	Drowsiness. Potentiates other sedatives. Confusion. Blurred vision. Bradycardia.
Metoclopramide	Dystonic reactions — particularly in children.

CARDIOVASCULAR SYSTEM

HEART

Cardiac Glycosides	
Digitalis Digoxin	Anorexia, nausea, vomiting. Fatigue and muscular weakness. Confusion. Visual disturbances—yellow or green vision.

	Arrhythmias — all types but most common are coupled ventricular extrasystoles, atrial tachycardia with A-V block, and first and second degree heart block.
	Toxicity enhanced in the elderly, renal failure, hypothyroidism, and by hypokalaemia or hypercalcaemia.
Anti-arrhythmic Drugs	
Quinidine Procainamide	Cardiac failure. Hypotension. Ventricular arrhythmias. DLE syndrome — (procainamide).
Lignocaine	Hypotension. Twitching and convulsions.
β-blockers	
Propranolol Practolol Oxprenolol	Bradycardia, cardiac failure, hypotension. Bronchospasm—more likely to occur with propranolol and oxprenolol. Practolol produces psoriasiform rashes, conjunctival scarring, corneal opacities, positive LE cells and ANF, and fibrous peritonitis.
Vasodilators	
Glyceryl Trinitrate	Headache, flushing, dizziness.

ANTIHYPERTENSIVE DRUGS

Guanethidine **Bethanidine**	Postural hypotension. Failure of ejaculation.

Debrisoquine	Diarrhoea — especially with guanethidine.
Reserpine	Depression. Nasal stuffiness. Dry mouth. Diarrhoea. Bradycardia.
Methyldopa	Tiredness. Depression. Fever. Diarrhoea. Fluid retention. Failure of ejaculation—uncommon. Positive Coombs' test (may interfere with cross-matching of blood for transfusion). Haemolytic anaemia — uncommon.
Clonidine	Tiredness. Depression. Fluid retention. Dry mouth. Constipation. Sudden withdrawal may produce severe hypertension.
Diazoxide	Fluid retention. Hyperglycaemia. Flushing. Diabetes and hirsutism may occur after prolonged use.
Hydrallazine	Headache. Flushing. Palpitation. Positive ANF and DLE syndrome.
Pentolinium	Blurred vision. Paralytic ileus. Urinary retention.

DIURETICS

Thiazides	
Bendrofluazide Chlorothiazide Hydroflumethiazide Chlorthalidone	Hypokalaemia. Potentiation of digoxin. Hyperuricaemia and occasionally gout. Hyperglycaemia and diabetes. Acute retention of urine. May precipitate coma in hepatic failure. Rashes. Thrombocytopenia.
Frusemide **Ethacrynic Acid**	As for thiazides but less risk of diabetes. Rapid I.V. injection may produce deafness, especially in renal failure.
Spironolactone	Hyperkalaemia. Gynaecomastia.
Amiloride **Triamterene**	Hyperkalaemia.
Enteric coated diuretics with potassium salts	Small bowel ulceration and stenosis.

ANTI-COAGULANTS

	May cause haemorrhage. Dosage needs careful adjustment with laboratory control for oral anti-coagulants.
Heparin	Hypersensitivity reactions: Urticaria, rhinitis, alopecia.
Coumarins	
Warfarin Dicoumarol Nicoumalone	Neonatal haemorrhage if used in last two weeks of pregnancy.

	Haemorrhagic skin necrosis. Alopecia. Many drug interactions (See Appendix IV).
Phenindione	Hypersensitivity reactions: rashes, fever, diarrhoea, jaundice, proteinuria, nephropathy. Alopecia. Orange-red urine.

LIPID METABOLISM

Cholestyramine	Constipation. Hypoprothrombinaemia due to malabsorption of Vitamin K. Interferes with absorption of other drugs, e.g. thyroxine, warfarin.
Clofibrate (Atromid S)	Muscle pain and stiffness associated with increased serum transaminases and creatinine phosphokinase.

RESPIRATORY SYSTEM

Iodides: in many cough mixtures	Hypersensitivity reactions: anaphylaxis, rashes. Iodism. Interfere with thyroid function tests. Hypothyroidism.

DRUGS USED TO RELIEVE BRONCHOSPASM

Adrenaline	Tachycardia. Arrhythmias. Hypertension. Tremor.

Isoprenaline **Orciprenaline**	Tachycardia. Arrhythmias. Tremor. Excessive use of isoprenaline aerosols may cause sudden death.
Salbutamol **Terbutaline**	Relatively selective for bronchial receptors. Cardiac effects less likely to occur.
Ephedrine	Urinary retention. Insomnia. Psychosis. Tremor.
Aminophylline — I.V. **— oral**	Tachycardia. Hypotension. Convulsions. Nausea.
Beclomethasone Dipropionate	Pharyngeal and laryngeal candidiasis if doses greater than 200 μg/day given for prolonged treatment.

RESPIRATORY STIMULANTS

Nikethamide **Doxapram, etc.**	Restlessness. Convulsions. Itching.
OXYGEN	CO_2 retention in respiratory insufficiency.

NERVOUS SYSTEM

ANALGESICS

Aspirin and Salicylates	Gastric irritation, gastrointestinal bleeding. Impaired haemostasis. Hypoprothrombinaemia. Iron deficiency anaemia. Hypersensitivity rashes. Urticaria.

	Bronchospasm in predisposed individuals. Tinnitus. May contribute to analgesic nephropathy.
Phenacetin	Analgesic nephropathy. Methaemoglobinaemia. Haemolytic anaemia.
Paracetamol	May contribute to analgesic nephropathy. Overdose may produce fatal hepatic necrosis.
Phenylbutazone and Oxyphenbutazone	Peptic ulceration. Hypersensitivity reactions: rashes, fever, jaundice, salivary gland swelling. Agranulocytosis and aplastic anaemia. Fluid retention and oedema.
Indomethacin	Nausea. Peptic ulceration. Headache. Depression. Rashes. Fluid retention. Corneal and retinal damage.
Ibuprofen **Mefenamic Acid** **Flufenamic Acid** **Naproxen**	Peptic ulceration.
Narcotic Analgesics	
Morphine Heroin Pethidine	Drug dependence. Respiratory depression. Nausea and vomiting. Constipation (morphine and heroin). Hypotension.

Pentazocine	Nausea, vomiting, dizziness. Dysphoria, confusion, hallucinations. Respiratory depression. Drug dependence uncommon. Withdrawal symptoms if given to opiate addicts.

HYPNOTICS AND SEDATIVES

All may produce respiratory depression in patients with impaired respiratory function.

Barbiturates	Tolerance. Dependence. Withdrawal syndrome of insomnia, anxiety and convulsions. Confusion in the elderly. Respiratory depression. Potentiated by alcohol and other CNS depressants. Rashes. [Blood dyscrasias] Porphyria in susceptible individuals.
Mandrax (Methaqualone and Diphenhydramine)	Dependence. Abuse. Potentiated by alcohol and other CNS depressants.
Benzodiazepines	
Nitrazepam Diazepam Chlordiazepoxide Oxazepam	Ataxia, dizziness, hypotension especially in the elderly. Potentiated by alcohol and other CNS depressants. Dependence can occur.

TRANQUILLISERS

Phenothiazines	
Chlorpromazine Promazine Thioridazine Trifluoperazine Fluphenazine	Parkinsonism — dystonic reactions. Akathisia (= restlessness). Cholestatic jaundice. Cardiac arrhythmias. Hypotension. Skin pigmentation. Photosensitivity. Corneal and lens opacities. Retinal pigmentation. Agranulocytosis. Depression.
Haloperidol **Trifluperidol**	Extrapyramidal syndromes and severe dystonic reactions common.

ANTI-DEPRESSANTS

Tricyclic Anti-depressants	
Imipramine Amitriptyline Nortriptyline	Postural hypotension, palpitations, cardiac arrhythmias. Anticholinergic effects, e.g. dry mouth, urinary retention, constipation. Tremor. Fluid retention.
Monoamine Oxidase Inhibitors	
Phenelzine Iproniazid Nialamide Isocarboxazid Tranylcypromine	Jaundice. Anticholinergic effects. Postural hypotension. Hypertensive crisis with severe headache and risk of

	subarachnoid haemorrhage, due to interaction with food, e.g. cheese, bovril; or with other drugs (see under drug interactions).
LITHIUM CARBONATE	Anorexia, Diarrhoea, Polyuria & polydipsia, Tremor, Muscle Weakness — Dose-related Goitre and hypothyroidism with prolonged use. Leucocytosis.
ANTICONVULSANTS	
Phenytoin **Methoin** **Ethotoin**	Nystagmus, dizziness, ataxia· Long term effects: Hyperplasia of gums. Folate deficiency and megaloblastic anaemia. Hypocalcaemia and osteomalacia. Hypersensitivity reactions: Rashes, DLE syndrome. [Lymphadenopathy]
Phenobarbitone **Primidone**	Nystagmus, dizziness, ataxia. Long term effects: Folate deficiency and megaloblastic anaemia. Hypocalcaemia and osteomalacia. Hypersensitivity rashes. Porphyria.

	Stimulation of hepatic microsomal enzymes (see drug interactions).
Sulthiame	Drowsiness, giddiness, ataxia. Hyperventilation, paraesthesiae.
Troxidone **Paramethadione**	Photophobia. Hiccups. Rashes. Blood dyscrasias. Nephrotic syndrome.
Ethosuximide	Vomiting. Hiccups. Rashes.
Carbamazepine	Drowsiness, dizziness, ataxia. Nausea, vomiting. Hypersensitivity reactions common — rashes, blood dyscrasias.

ANTI-PARKINSON DRUGS

L-Dopa	Nausea and vomiting. Postural hypotension. Dystonic reactions. Dyskinesias. Psychoses. Confusion. Nightmares (all dose related). Positive Coombs Test.
Benzhexol **Benztropine** **Orphenadrine** **Procyclidine**	Confusional states. Atropine-like effects: Dry mouth. Constipation. Urinary retention.

MUSCLE RELAXANTS

Tubocurarine **Gallamine** **Pancuronium**	Myasthenic patients very sensitive. Bronchospasm, vasodilatation and hypotension (tubocurarine).

Suxamethonium	Muscle pain.
	Bradycardia and arrhythmias.
	Allergic reactions — bronchospasm.
	Prolonged effect in severe liver disease and hereditary psuedocholinesterase deficiency.
	Malignant hyperpyrexia in susceptible patients.

ANAESTHETICS

All anaesthetics produce vasodilatation and hypotension. The respiratory centre is depressed by anaesthesia; this may be dangerous in patients with raised intracranial pressure.

Inhalation Agents	
Cyclopropane	Cardiac arrhythmias.
Ether	Post-operative vomiting.
Halothane	Cardiac arrhythmias.
	Jaundice — especially if administration repeated at short intervals.
Methoxyflurane	Polyuric renal failure.
	Jaundice.
Trichlorethylene	Cardiac arrhythmias.
Intravenous Anaesthetics	
Thiopentone Methohexitone	Local irritation if injected outside vein:
	Arterial thrombosis and gangrene.
	Nerve palsies.
	Laryngospasm.
	Porphyria in predisposed individuals.
	Methohexitone may produce convulsions in susceptible patients.

Ketamine	Hypertension. Confusional states and unpleasant "dreams" during recovery.
Propanidid	Hypotension greater than with barbiturates. Hypersensitivity reactions.

LOCAL ANAESTHETICS

Cocaine	Cerebral stimulation. Convulsions. Respiratory depression. Myocardial depression. Circulatory failure. Drug dependence.
Amethocaine **Bupivicaine** **Benzocaine** **Lignocaine** **Prilocaine** **Procaine**	Systemic toxicity as for cocaine. Skin sensitisation. Contact dermatitis. Methaemoglobinaemia (procaine and prilocaine).
Vasoconstrictors	
Adrenaline Noradrenaline	Tachycardia and arrhythmias. Hypertension.

GENITAL SYSTEM

SEX HORMONES

Androgens	
Methyltestosterone Testosterone oenanthate Anabolic agents: Methandienone Nandrolone Norethandronlone Oxymethalone	Cholestatic jaundice. Oedema. Virilisation in women. Precocious sexual development in boys. Accelerated bone maturation in children.

Oestrogens

Stilboestrol Ethinyloestradiol	Nausea, headache, fluid retention. Thrombosis and thromboembolism. Used in women: Withdrawal bleeding. Postmenopausal bleeding. Used in men: Gynaecomastia and loss of libido.

ORAL CONTRACEPTIVES

Oestrogens

Ethinyloestradiol Mestranol **Progestagens** Norethisterone Lynoestrenol Megestrol Ethynodial Norethynodrel Chlormadinone	Nausea. Headache. Fluid retention and weight gain. Hypertension. Depression, loss of libido (?). Genital candidiasis. Jaundice (rare). Amenorrhoea may persist after stopping pill. May precipitate porphyria in susceptible individuals. Increased risk of thrombosis and thromboembolism. PBI elevated due to increased thyroid binding globulin.

INFECTIONS

ANTIBACTERIAL DRUGS

Penicillins

Ampicillin Benzylpenicillin Cloxacillin Carbenicillin Methicillin Phenethicillin Phenoxymethylpenicillin Procaine Penicillin	All cause hypersensitivity reactions. Anaphylaxis and angioneurotic oedema more likely after parenteral administration. If patient is sensitive to one penicillin he is usually sensitive to all. Ampicillin produces rashes, not due to sensitivity, particularly in patients with infectious mononucleosis. Large I.V. doses of benzylpenicillin or carbenicillin may produce convulsions, hypokalaemia and (rarely) haemolytic anaemia.

Cephalosporins

Cephaloridine Cephatholin Cephalexin	Hypersensitivity rashes and fever. Cross-sensitivity to penicillin occurs — rarely. Large doses of cephaloridine are nephrotoxic.

Tetracyclines

Demethylchlortetracycline Chlortetracycline Doxycycline Lymecycline Oxytetracycline Tetracycline	Gastrointestinal irritation. Diarrhoea. Superinfection with resistant organisms—candida, staphylococci, pseudomonas. Increase blood urea in patients with impaired renal function.

	May reduce glomerular filtration rate. Chelate with calcium and are deposited in bones and teeth of fetus and children under 7 yrs. Demethyltetracycline produces skin photosensitivity. [Jaundice — high doses IV in pregnancy.]
Chloramphenicol	Reversible bone marrow depression common. Aplastic anaemia rare but usually fatal. Circulatory failure (grey syndrome) in neonates.
Aminoglycosides	
Streptomycin Dihydrostreptomycin (obsolete) Gentamicin Kanamycin Neomycin	Ototoxicity. Nephrotoxicity. Neuromuscular blockade and aggravation of myasthenia gravis. Risk of toxicity greater in patients with impaired renal function. Skin sensitisation common with topical use. Neomycin may produce a malabsorption syndrome.
Polymixins	
Colistin Polymixin B	Nephrotoxicity. Ototoxicity. Dizziness and circumoral paraesthesiae. Neuromuscular blockade.

Lincomycin, Clindamycin	Diarrhoea. Pseudomembranous colitis.
Erythromycin Estolate	Jaundice. Abdominal pain.
Vancomycin	Ototoxicity. Thrombophlebitis.
Novobiocin	Jaundice — particularly in neonates.
Nitrofurantoin	Nausea. Rashes and fever. Peripheral neuropathy — especially if renal function is impaired. Hypersensitivity pneumonitis. Haemolytic anaemia.
Nalidixic acid	Rashes. Photosensitivity. Haemolytic anaemia. Raised intracranial pressure and papilloedema in children.
Sulphonamides	Hypersensitivity reactions: Rashes — especially if applied topically. Photosensitivity. Fever. Erythema nodosum. Polyarteritis nodosa. Stevens-Johnson syndrome. Blood dyscrasias. Crystalluria — especially sulphadiazine.
Co-trimoxazole (sulphamethoxazole + trimethoprim)	As for sulphonamides. Trimethoprim may interfere with folate metabolism, but megaloblastic haemopoiesis is very uncommon.

Sulphasalazine	Nausea. Hypersensitivity reactions.

ANTI-TUBERCULOUS DRUGS

Streptomycin	See under aminoglycosides (p. 142).
p-Aminosalicylic acid	Gastric irritation. Hypersensitivity reactions—rashes, fever, jaundice, lymphadenopathy. Goitre.
Isoniazid	Peripheral neuropathy — corrected by pyridoxine. Pellagra-like syndrome. Positive antinuclear factor and DLE syndrome. Jaundice.
Ethionamide **Prothionamide**	High incidence of toxicity. Nausea and vomiting. Jaundice. Hypersensitivity, rashes and fever. Acne, Pigmentation. Alopecia. Headache, giddiness, depression, paraesthesiae.
Pyrazinamide	Nausea and vomiting. Hyperuricaemia — gout. Jaundice.
Cycloserine	Neurotoxicity.
Ethambutol	Optic neuritis (retrobulbar). Loss of yellow-green colour vision.

Thiacetazone	Hypersensitivity rashes. Agranulocytosis. Haemolytic anaemia.
Rifampicin	Jaundice. Nephritis. Immune thrombocytopenia. Colours urine, sputum and tears red.

LEPROSY

Dapsone	Dose-related haemolytic anaemia. Hypersensitivity rashes. Erythema nodosum.

ANTI-FUNGAL DRUGS

Griseofulvin	Porphyria in susceptible individuals.
Amphotericin B	Nephrotoxic. Normochromic anaemia. Hypokalaemia. Thrombophlebitis at injection site.

ANTIMALARIAL DRUGS

Chloroquine	Retinal and corneal damage. Myopathy. Skin photosensitivity. Exacerbation of cutaneous porphyria.
Primaquine	Haemolytic anaemia in G-6-PD deficiency.
Pyrimethamine	Interferes with folate metabolism. Blood dyscrasias.

Mepacrine	Yellow pigmentation of skin. Aplastic anaemia.
Quinine	Hypersensitivity reactions—immune thrombocytopenia. Optic atrophy. Ototoxicity.

ANTI-AMOEBIC

Emetine	Nausea. Myocarditis.

TRYPANOCIDES

Pentamidine	Sudden hypotension after rapid injection. Hypoglycaemia. Diabetes.
Suramin	Nephrotoxic. Proteinuria.

ANTHELMINTICS

Stibophen	Haemolytic anaemia.
Antimony Sodium Tartrate	Toxic effects on heart.
Lucanthone	Vomiting. Headache. Convulsions. Psychosis.
Niridazole	Toxic effects on heart. Vomiting. Headache. Convulsions. Drowsiness. Confusion. Allergic pneumonitis.
Male fern	Nausea, vomiting, abdominal cramp. Headache. Convulsions. Optic neuritis. Hyperbilirubinaemia. Proteinuria.

Piperazine	Neurotoxic in children, convulsions. Nausea, Diarrhoea. Urticaria.
Bephenium	Nausea. Diarrhoea.

MISCELLANEOUS

Clioquinol	Subacute myelo-optic neuropathy (SMON).

METABOLISM

CORTICOSTEROIDS

Cortisone **Hydrocortisone** **Prednisolone** **Prednisone,** **Fludrocortisone** **Dexamethazone** **Betamethazone**	Sodium retention. Hypertension. Potassium loss. Muscle weakness and wasting. Skin atrophy, striae, purpura, acne. Osteoporosis. Diabetes. Increased susceptibility to infection, reactivation of latent Tb, unusual infections. Reactivation of peptic ulcer. Cataracts. Glaucoma. Mental disturbances: Euphoria, depression, psychosis. Long term effects: Growth retardation in children.

	Adrenal atrophy and adrenal insufficiency. Hypotension during anaesthesia and infection.

CORTICOTROPHINS

ACTH **Tetracosactrin**	All effects of corticosteroids except adrenal atrophy. Allergic reactions.

ANABOLIC STEROIDS

(see Sex Hormones, pages 139–140)

DRUGS USED IN DIABETES

Insulin	Hypoglycaemia. Hypersensitivity reactions. Insulin resistance (May be specific to beef or pig insulins.) Lipoatrophy at injection sites.
Sulphonylureas	
Chlorpropamide Tolbutamide Glibenclamide	Hypoglycaemia — may be prolonged. Sulphonamide-like hypersensitivity reactions. Alcohol intolerance. Hypothyroidism.
Biguanides	
Phenformin Metformin	Lactic acidosis. Nausea and anorexia. Malabsorption of vitamin B_{12}.

DRUGS USED IN THYROID DISEASE

Thyroxine	May induce angina.
Antithyroid drugs	
Carbimazole Methylthiouracil Propylthiouracil	Hypersensitivity reactions: Rashes, fever. Agranulocytosis. Alopecia.
Potassium Perchlorate	Agranulocytosis. Aplastic anaemia.
Radioactive Iodine	Hypothyroidism. Possible risk of thyroid carcinoma.

STIMULANTS AND APPETITE SUPPRESSANTS

Amphetamines **Phenmetrazine** **Diethylpropion**	Dependence and withdrawal symptoms. Confusional states. Paranoid psychoses.
Fenfluramine	Drowsiness and lethargy. Diarrhoea. Nausea. Impotence. Withdrawal insomnia and depression.

LIPID METABOLISM

(See under Cardiovascular System, p. 131)

MALIGNANT DISEASE

General effects	Marrow depression: Leukopenia, thrombocytopenia. Aplastic anaemia. Mucosal ulceration: Stomatitis, nausea, vomiting and diarrhoea. Secondary infection.

Busulphan	Sudden fatal aplastic anaemia. Skin pigmentation. Pulmonary fibrosis.
Cyclophosphamide	Alopecia. Haemorrhagic cystitis. Testicular atrophy. Amenorrhoea.
Mercaptopurine	Jaundice.
Methotrexate	Alopecia. Hepatocellular necrosis. Pneumonitis.
Vincristine	Alopecia. Constipation and abdominal pain. Peripheral sensory and motor neuropathy. Hyponatraemia syndrome.
Actinomycin D	Alopecia.
Daunorubicin	Myocardial damage.

IMMUNOSUPPRESSANTS

Azathioprine	Marrow depression — anaemia, leucopenia and thrombocytopenia. Nausea. Hepatitis. Lowered resistance to infection. Lymphomas.
Antilymphocyte serum	Allergic reactions.

VITAMINS AND MINERALS

Vitamin D **Calciferol** (N.B. Calciferol tablets,	High doses can cause hypercalcaemia, renal calcification and renal failure.

strong BP contain 50,000 units of Vitamin D and should only be used in treatment of hypoparathyroidism and renal osteodystrophy)	
Vitamin K — water soluble analogues	May produce haemolysis and kernicterus in neonates.
Iron	
Oral iron tablets	Gastrointestinal irritation.
Intramuscular preparations Iron sorbitol	Skin staining. Pain. Headache, dizziness and vomiting.
Intravenous preparations Iron dextran	Anaphylactic reactions.

GOUT AND RHEUMATOID ARTHRITIS

Allopurinol	Hypersensitivity reactions: rashes, fever. May precipitate acute gout.
Probenecid	Rashes. [Nephrotic syndrome] May precipitate acute gout and renal colic.
Sulphinpyrazone	May precipitate acute gout and renal colic.
Colchicine	Nausea. Diarrhoea.
Gold Salts	Dermatitis. Skin pigmentation. Nephrotoxicity — proteinuria. Aplastic anaemia or thrombocytopenia. Stomatitis. Diarrhoea.

Chloroquine	See under Malaria (p. 145).
Penicillamine	Nausea. Loss of taste. Rashes. Thrombocytopenia, neutropenia. Proteinuria.

DRUGS ACTING ON MOUTH AND THROAT

Antiseptic lozenges	Sore mouth and ulceration.
Anaesthetic lozenges	Sensitivity reactions.

DRUGS ACTING ON THE EYE (Topical)

Eye drops and ointments	Bacterial contamination easily occurs and may be a serious hazard.
Corticosteroids	May precipitate glaucoma in susceptible individuals. Cataracts (prolonged use). Aggravate corneal ulceration due to herpes simplex and may cause blindness.
Antibacterial drugs	Sensitisation (particularly neomycin and sulphonamides).
Atropine **Cyclopentolate**	Action of atropine lasts up to a week. May precipitate glaucoma in predisposed individuals. Systemic absorption may produce confusion, hallucinations and hyperpyrexia.

Echothiopate	Systemic absorption may increase sensitivity to suxamethonium. Effect persists for many weeks. Cataract.
Physostigmine	May be painful.
Phenylephrine	Systemic absorption may produce tachycardia and hypertension. May produce hypertensive crisis in patients on MAOI.
Cocaine	May precipitate glaucoma in predisposed individuals. Damages corneal epithelium.
Pilocarpine	Cataract.

DRUGS USED ON THE SKIN

See drugs causing Contact Dermatitis (Appendix II)

Tar preparations	Photosensitivity.
Local Anaesthetics **Antihistamines** **Antibacterial drugs** Neomycin Streptomycin Penicillin Chlorpromazine **Other components ("vehicles")**	Skin sensitisation.
Corticosteroids	Systemic absorption may produce systemic side effects and adrenal suppression. Skin atrophy.

	Telangiectases in patients with rosacea — mainly with fluorinated ones. Infection and impaired healing of varicose ulcers.

VACCINES AND RELATED PRODUCTS

Cholera vaccine	Fever, headache, malaise. Local reactions — mild.
Measles vaccine (live, attenuated)	Mild measles-like illness. Encephalitis — rarely.
Measles vaccine (inactivated)	Mild measles-like illness. Several local reactions may occur during a subsequent natural measles infection.
Poliomyelitis vaccine (oral)	Diarrhoea.
Rubella vaccine (live, attenuated)	Mild rubella-like illness in adults. Intrauterine infection. Should not be given to pregnant women. Arthritis.
Smallpox vaccine	Local and generalised vaccinia. Should not be given to children with eczema. Post-vaccinal encephalomyelitis. Intrauterine infection. Should not be given to pregnant women.
Typhoid vaccine (TAB)	Fever and headache. Severe local reactions.

Antisera—Tetanus **Diphtheria**	Anaphylaxis, serum sickness.
Pertussis vaccine (usually given as triple vaccine)	Convulsions may occur rarely but a causal relationship has not been established.

APPENDIX II

DRUG INDUCED DISEASE

These lists are arranged under body systems as in Appendix I. Although most of the important drugs causing particular disorders are included, the lists are not comprehensive. Further information can be found in the references listed at the end of this appendix.

ALIMENTARY SYSTEM

(For drugs affecting the mouth and teeth see Chapter 5)

Nausea and vomiting	Digitalis. Narcotic analgesics. L-dopa. Cytotoxic drugs. Biguanides. p-Aminosalicylic acid, ethionamide. Oral iron preparations. (Many others.)
Gastric bleeding	Aspirin. Alcohol—potentiates aspirin.
Peptic ulceration	Phenylbutazone, oxyphenbutazone. Indomethacin. Flufenamic acid, mefenamic acid. Ibuprofen, naproxen. Corticosteroids — high doses
Small bowel ulceration and stenosis	Enteric coated potassium salts. (Slow release forms probably not hazardous.)

Malabsorption/Steatorrhoea	Neomycin. Colchicine. p-Aminosalicylic acid. Biguanides malabsorption Vitamin B_{12}. Cholestyramine.
Diarrhoea	Guanethidine, methyldopa. Broad spectrum antibiotics. Lincomycin, clindamycin — (pseudomembranous colitis). Colchicine. Cytotoxic drugs. Laxative abuse.
Constipation	Ganglion blockers. Anticholinergic drugs: Atropine. Anti-Parkinsonism drugs. Tricyclic antidepressants. Phenothiazines. Clonidine. Morphine, codeine, dihydrocodeine.
Jaundice	Interference with bilirubin uptake or conjugation: Rifampicin Novobiocin. Dose-related cholestasis: Methyltestosterone. Norethandrolone Direct hepatotoxicity: Methotrexate, mercaptopurine, azathioprine. Paracetamol overdose. Hepatitis-like reactions: Halothane — especially

after repeated administration.
Rifampicin. Isoniazid.
Methyldopa.
MAOIs — iproniazid, isocarboxazid, phenelzine.
Oxyphenisatin — a constituent of many proprietary laxatives.

Cholestatis ± hepatitis:
Chlorpromazine and other phenothizines.
Tricyclic antidepressants — iprindole, amitriptyline, imipramine.
Pyrazinamide.
Chlorpropamide.
Phenylbutazone.
Oral contraceptives (very rare — probable genetic basis).

Hepatic coma precipitated by: Diuretics — Thiazides
Frusemide
Ethacrynicacid.
Sedatives and Hypnotics.
Narcotic analgesics.

CARDIOVASCULAR SYSTEM

Cardiac Arrhythmias
Digitalis.
Quinidine, procainamide.
Adrenaline, isoprenaline.
Atropine.
Phenothiazines — especially thioridazine.
Tricyclic antidepressants.
L-dopa.

Hypertension	Oral contraceptives. Corticosteroids. Carbenoxolone. MAOIs together with sympathomimetic amines (see appendix III).
Direct Myocardial Toxicity	Emetine. Daunorubicin. Phenothiazines.
Anaphylactic shock	Penicillins. Intravenous iron (iron dextran). Antisera. Dextrans. Streptokinase.

RESPIRATORY SYSTEM

Pulmonary fibrosis	Busulphan. Cyclophosphamide. Methysergide. Radiation. Prolonged high-dose oxygen therapy.
Allergic pneumonitis	Nitrofurantoin. Methotrexate. Sulphonamides. PAS. Niridazole.
Bronchospam in predisposed individuals (see also Anaphylaxis)	Tubocurarine. Carbachol. Propranolol, oxprenolol, (practolol — rarely). Aspirin and other analgesics.

Pulmonary oedema	Heroin overdose.
Pulmonary embolism	Oral contraceptives.
Respiratory depression	Narcotic analgesics. All hypnotics and sedatives. Diphenoxylate (Lomotil). Oxygen in chronic respiratory disease.
2° Pulmonary infection	Broad-spectrum antibiotics. Cytotoxic drugs. Immunosuppressants. Corticosteroids.
Lipid pneumonia	Bronchography. Lymphography. Mineral oil inhalation.

NERVOUS SYSTEM

Headache	Indomethacin.
Cerebral thrombosis	Oral contraceptives.
Confusional states — most likely to occur in elderly patients	Hypnotics and sedatives e.g. barbiturates nitrazepam diazepam. Antidepressants. Atropine, hyoscine. Antiparkinsonism drugs e.g. benzhexol benztropine amantidine l-dopa. Pentazocine. Digitalis. Isoniazid, ethionamide, cycloserine.

Depression	Antihypertensive drugs —reserpine methyldopa clonidine.
	Corticosteroids.
	Indomethacin.
	Phenothiazines.
	L-dopa.
	Fenfluramine — after withdrawal.
Psychotic reactions	LSD.
	Amphetamines.
	L-dopa.
	Corticosteroids.
	Isoniazid, ethionamide, cycloserine.
Drug dependence	Narcotic analgesics.
	Barbiturates — and other hypnotics.
	Chlordiazepoxide, diazepam.
	Amphetamines.
	Phenacetin.
Convulsions	Phenothiazines.
	Tricyclic antidepressants.
	Methohexitone.
	Lignocaine. Local anaesthetics.
	Cycloserine.
	Vaccines.
	Drug dependence — withdrawal of e.g. alcohol, barbiturates and other hypnotics.

Extrapyramidal syndromes Parkinsonism Dystonic reactions	Phenothiazines. Butyrophenones. L-dopa. Metoclopramide — especially in children.
Peripheral neuropathy	Isoniazid. Ethionamide. Cycloserine. Nitrofurantoin. Clioquinol. Vincristine. Thalidomide.
Myasthenic Syndrome (Neuromuscular block)	Streptomycin, neomycin, kanamycin, gentamicin, colistin, polymixin B. Quinidine.
Myopathy (see also : Hypokalaemia Osteomalacia)	Corticosteroids. Chloroquine.
Muscle pain	Suxamethonium. Clofibrate. Bumetaride (used in renal failure).

EYE

Corneal opacities	Phenothiazines. Chloroquine. Indomethacin. Corticosteroids. Practolol.
Corneal ulceration	Corticosteroid eye drops — aggravation of herpes simplex keratitis.
Cataract	Corticosteriods — local or systemic. Chlorpromazine. Piperazine. Eclothiopate iodide eyedrops.

Glaucoma	Corticosteroids Atropine. Propantheline. Benzhexol, benztropine, orphenadrine. Tricyclic antidepressants. Mydriatic eye drops— atropine homatropine adrenaline.
Retinal damage	Chloroquine. Phenothiazines — e.g. thioridazine chlorpromazine. Indomethacin.
Optic neuritis **Optic atrophy** **Toxic amblyopia**	Quinine. Organic arsenicals. Clioquinol. Chloramphenicol. Ethambutol. Ethionamide. Cycloserine.
Disturbances of colour vision	Digitalis. Ethambutol.
Photophobia	Troxidone.
Nystagmus	Barbiturates and other hypnotics. Phenytoin.
Papilloedema and raised intracranial pressure	Corticosteroids — especially in children. Nalidixic acid — especially in children. Tetracyclines. Oral contraceptives.

EAR

Deafness and/or vertigo	Aminoglycoside antibiotics: neomycin, kanamycin, streptomycin, dihydrostreptomycin, gentamicin. Salicylates. Quinine and quindine. Ethacrynic acid } Rapid IV Frusemide } injection

LOCOMOTOR SYSTEM

Osteoporosis	Corticosteroids. Heparin (long term).
Osteomalacia	Anticonvulsants.
Arthralgia or Arthritis	Antisera. Penicillin. p-Aminosalicylic acid. Iron dextran. Live attenuated Rubella vaccine.
DLE syndrome	Hydralazine. Isoniazid. Procainamide. Phenytoin — and other hydantoins. (Occasional reports with many other drugs.)
Serum Sickness	Antisera. Penicillin. Sulphonamides. Thiouracils.

GENITO-URINARY SYSTEM

Direct nephrotoxicity — Acute renal failure	Neomycin, kanamycin (rare with other aminoglycosides). Colistin. Cephaloridine. Amphotericin B. Hypervitaminosis D (hypercalcaemia).
Acute polyuric renal failure	Methoxyflurane.
Crystalluria and acute renal failure	Sulphonamides.
Hypersensitivity nephritis Proteinuria Nephrotic syndrome (see also: Serum sickness DLE syndrome)	Sulphonamides. Penicillins. Phenindione. Troxidone. Gold salts. Penicillamine. Rifampicin. Probenecid.
Chronic interstitial fibrosis ("Analgesic Nephropathy")	Compound analgesic preparations. These usually contain phenacetin, but aspirin and other analgesics may also be responsible.
Rise in blood urea due to anti-anabolic effect. Deterioration in renal function in patients with chronic renal failure	Tetracyclines.
Retroperitoneal fibrosis and obstructive uropathy	Methysergide.
Urinary retention	Ephedrine. Antidepressants.
Failure of ejaculation	Antihypertensive drugs.

ENDOCRINE AND METABOLIC DISORDERS

Hypothyroidism	I^{131}. Iodides. Antithyroid drugs— carbimazole thiouracil. p-Aminosalicylic acid, ethionamide. Phenylbutazone. Lithium. Sulphonylureas. (Phenytoin lowers PBI by displacing thyroxine from protein-binding.)
Amenorrhoea	Oral contraceptives. Cyclophosphamide. Phenothiazines.
Infertility	Cyclophosphamide. Chlorambucil.
Gynaecomastia	Oestrogens. Spironolactone. Digitalis.
Galactorrhoea	Phenothiazines, haloperidol. Imipramine. Reserpine. Methyldopa.
Porphyria — exacerbations in susceptible subjects	Barbiturates. Griseofulvin. Dichloralphenazone. Sulphonylureas. Oral contraceptives. Chloroquine (cutaneous form only).

Hyperuricaemia ± gout	Cytotoxic drugs. Diuretics — thiazides, chlorthalidone, frusemide, ethacrynic acid. Pyrazinamide.
Hyperglycaemia	Corticosteroids. Diuretics — thiazides, chlorthalidone, frusemide, ethacrynic acid. Diazoxide. Oral contraceptives (mild impairment of glucose tolerance test).
Hypoglycaemia	Insulin. Sulphonylureas. Propranolol may prolong hypoglycaemia produced by insulin or sulphonylureas.
Oedema	Corticosteroids. Oral contraceptives. Carbenoxolone. Phenylbutazone, oxyphenbutazone, indomethacin. Guanethidine, methyldopa, clonidine, reserpine. Diazoxide.
Hypokalaemia	Diuretics — thiazides, frusemide, ethacrynic acid. Carbenoxolone. Laxative abuse. Carbenicillin (large doses). Amphotericin B. Corticosteroids.

Hyperkalaemia	Triamterene. Spironolactone. Amiloride.
Water intoxication	Chlorpropamide. Cyclophosphamide. Vincristine.
Diabetes insipidus	Lithium.
Lactic acidosis	Biguanides.

BLOOD DISEASES

Hypochromic anaemia due to Gastrointestinal bleeding	Aspirin. Indomethacin. Phenylbutazone, oxyphenbutazone. Alcohol — potentiates bleeding due to aspirin.
Megaloblastic anaemia	Anticonvulsants. Methotrexate, cytosine, arabinoside. Triamterene. Pyrimethamine. Trimethoprim. Oral contraceptives (doubtful).
Haemolytic anaemia	
Mainly in G6PD deficiency	Primaquine.
Large doses in normal individuals.	Sulphonamides. Dapsone (occurs in normal individuals at therapeutic doses). Nitrofurantoin. Phenacetin.
Immune mechanism	Stibophen. Phenacetin. Quinine, quinidine.

	p-Aminosalicylic acid Rifampicin. Methyldopa. Penicillin (large doses). Cephalosporins.
Aplastic anaemia	Cytotoxic drugs. Chloramphenicol. Phenylbutazone, oxyphenbutazone. Indomethacin. Sulphonamides. Sulphonylureas. Diphenylhydantoin. Trimethadione. Ethosuximide. Carbamazepine. Antithyroid drugs. Gold. Mepacrine. Meprobamate. Amidopyrine, Phenothiazines } Usually produce isolated agranulocytosis.
Thrombocytopenia	Drugs producing aplastic anaemia may produce isolated thrombocytopenia. Others: Thiazide diuretics, frusemide. Penicillinamine. Co-trimoxazole. Rifampicin. Quinine, quinidine. Antazoline.
Leucocytosis	Lithium carbonate.

Methaemoglobinaemia	Phenacetin. Sulphonamides. Local anaesthetics.
Thromboembolism	Oestrogens. Oral contraceptives.

SKIN REACTIONS

The aetiology of most skin reactions is unknown. Some are the result of direct toxicity and are dose related, a few are known to be allergic, but many can only be labelled "idiosyncratic".

Almost any drug can affect the skin. Many skin reactions are entirely non-specific, and are produced by a wide variety of chemically and pharmacologically unrelated drugs. Furthermore, the same drug can produce different reactions in different patients.

It is, therefore, impossible to provide a comprehensive list of drugs producing each type of reaction. In the following tables a list of the drugs which most commonly affect the skin is given first, followed by those most likely to produce specific skin reactions.

Drugs which commonly produce skin reactions of several types	Penicillins. Aminoglycosides — streptomycin, neomycin. Sulphonamides, sulphones. Sulphonylureas. Thiazide diuretics. Barbiturates. Hydantoins e.g phenytoin. Phenothiazines. Phenylbutazone. Metal salts — gold, arsenic, bismuth. Cytotoxic drugs.

Urticaria	Penicillins. Aspirin. Barbiturates. Antitoxins. Iodine — X-ray contrast media.
Exanthematous Eruptions	Penicillins — especially ampicillin — high incidence in infectious mononucleosis. Sulphonamides. Thiazide diuretics, frusemide. Barbiturates. Hydantoins e.g. phenytoin. Phenothiazines, tricyclic antidepressants. Carbamazepine. Phenylbutazone. Gold salts. Streptomycin. p-Aminosalicylic acid. Nalidixic acid. Nitrofurantoin. Allopurinol. Phenindione.
Erythema multiforme **Stevens Johnson Syndrome**	Sulphonamides — especially long acting ones. Chlorpropamide. Barbiturates. Hydantoins e.g. phenytoin.
Erythema Nodosum	Sulphonamides. Penicillin. Dapsone. Oral contraceptives.
Psoriasiform rash	Practolol.

Fixed Eruptions	Phenolphthalein. Barbiturates. Phenacetin. Sulphonamides. Dapsone. Tetracyclines. Quinine.
Toxic Epidermal Necrolysis (Lyell's Syndrome)	Sulphonamides. Dapsone. Phenylbutazone. Hydantoins e.g. Phenytoin. Barbiturates.
Drug-Induced D.L.E.	See under Locomotor System (p. 164).
Contact Dermatitis	Topical application of many drugs — especially: Neomycin, streptomycin. Penicillins. Sulphonamides. Antihistamines. Phenothiazines. Local anaesthetics.
Exfoliative Dermatitis	Systemic use of drugs which have produced contact sensitisation. Also: Gold salts. Quinine, chloroquine. Sulphonamides. Phenylbutazone. Phenindione. Barbiturates. Carbamazepine.
Purpura	See under thrombocytopenia (p. 169). Non-thrombocytopenic: Carbromal.

	Meprobamate.
	Corticosteroids.
	Frusemide.
	Aspirin.
	Anticoagulants.
Pigmentation	Phenothiazines.
	Chloroquine, mepacrine.
	Busulfan.
	Phenytoin.
	Heavy metals — gold, arsenic.
	Oral contraceptives (Chloasma).
Light-induced Reactions	Phenothiazines.
	Sulphonamides.
	Sulphonylureas.
	Thiazide diuretics.
	Antihistamines.
	Demethylchlortetracycline.
	Griseofulvin.
	Nalidixic acid.
	Coal tar derivatives.
Alopecia	Cytotoxic drugs — especially cyclophosphamide.
	Antithyroid drugs — carbimazole.
	Anticoagulants — heparin and oral anticoagulants.
Acne	Corticosteroids and ACTH.
	Androgenic hormones (in women).
	Iodides, bromides.
	Isoniazid.
	Anticonvulsants — especially hydantoins.
	Ethionamide.

Hirsutism	Corticosteroids. Androgens. Diazoxide. Phenytoin.
Skin Atrophy and Striae	Corticosteroids.
Raynaud's Syndrome	Ergotamine. Propranolol. Clonidine.
Pruritis	Narcotic analgesics. Nikethamide and other respiratory stimulants. Drugs producing chloestatic jaundice. (Many rashes are accompanied or preceded by itching.)
Lichenoid Eruptions	Gold salts. Antimalarials — quinine, chloroquine. Phenothiazines. p-Aminosalicylic acid. Thiazide diuretics. Quinidine.
Bullous Eruptions	Drug-induced coma — especially barbiturates. Iodides, bromides. Salicylates. Penicillins. Sulphonamides.
Haemorrhagic Bullous Necrosis	Oral anticoagulants.

BIBLIOGRAPHY FOR APPENDIX II

General

Meyler, L. and Peck, H. M. (Ed.) (1972). Drug Induced diseases. Vol. 4. Excerpta Medica.

Meyler L. and Herxheimer, A. (Ed.) (1968). Side effects of drugs. Vol. 6. Excerpta Medica.

Meyler, L. and Herxheimer, A. (Ed.) (1972). Side effects of drugs. Vol. 7. Excerpta Medica.

Specific

Maxwell, J. D. and Williams, R. (1971). Adverse drug reactions and the liver. Adverse drug reaction bulletin, **29,** 84.

Feinmann, L. (1974). Drug induced lung disease. Adverse drug reaction bulletin, **45,** 148.

Leading Article. (1973). Drug induced respiratory disorders. Brit. Med. J., ii, 320.

McClelland, H. A. (1973). Psychiatric complications of drug therapy. Adverse drug reaction bulletin, **40,** 128.

Editorial. (1969). Drugs and the eye — Parts I and II. Adverse drug reaction bulletin, **17** and **18.**

Mushin, A. S. (1972). Ocular damage by drugs in children. Adverse drug reaction bulletin, **36,** 112.

Kerr, D. N. S. and Walls, J. (1970). Renal damage due to drugs. Adverse drug reaction bulletin, **20** and **21,** 54–59.

Evered, D. and Hall, R. (1972). Drugs and the endocrine system. Adverse drug reaction bulletin, **34,** 104.

Girdwood, R. H. (Ed.) (1973). Blood disorders due to drugs and other agents. Excerpta Medica.

Bruinsma, W. (1973). A guide to drug eruptions. Excerpta Medica.

Dower, Francis H. and Stevenson, C. J. (1973). Contact dermatitis from topical drugs. Adverse drug reaction bulletin, **42,** 136.

Baker, H. and Levene, G. M. (1969). Cutaneous reactions to anti-coagulants. Brit. J. Dermatol., **81,** 236.

Baker, H. and Moore-Robinson, M. (1970). Cutaneous responses to aspirin and its derivatives. Brit. J. Dermatol., **82,** 319.

Almeyda, J. and Baker. H. (1970). Adverse reactions to hypoglycaemic agents. Brit. J. Dermatol., **82,** 634.

Almeyda, J. and Baker, H. (1971). Cutaneous reactions to imipramine and chlordiazepoxide. Brit. J. Dermatol., **84,** 298.

Almeyda, J. and Levantine, A. (1971). Lichenoid drug eruptions. Brit. J. Dermatol., **85,** 604.

Almeyda, J. and Baker, H. (1971). Cutaneous reactions to anti-rheumatic drugs. Brit. J. Dermatol., **84,** 707.

Almeyda, J. and Levantine, A. (1972). Cutaneous reactions to barbiturates, chloral hydrate and its derivatives. Brit. J. Dermatol., **86,** 313.

Levantine, A. and Almeyda, J. (1972). Cutaneous reactions to antituberculous drugs. Brit. J. Dermatol., **86**, 651.

Levantine, A. and Almeyda, J. (1972). Cutaneous reactions to anticonvulsants. Brit. J. Dermatol., **87**, 646.

Almeyda, J. and Levantine, A. (1973). Cutaneous reactions to cardiovascular drugs. Brit. J. Dermatol., **88**, 313.

Levantine, A. and Almeyda, J. (1973). Drug-induced changes in pigmentation. Brit. J. Dermatol., **89**, 105.

Levantine, A. and Almeyda, J. (1973). Drug-induced alopecia. Brit. J. Dermatol., **89**, 549.

APPENDIX III

DRUG INTERACTION TABLES

The following tables are not comprehensive but contain most of those interactions which are known to be, or are likely to be important in man during normal clinical use of the drugs concerned. When using the tables it is important to be aware that interactions occurring with one member of a group of related drugs may also affect other members of the same group.

Many reviews and lists of drug interactions have been published recently (Hansten, 1973, APA, 1973, Stockley, 1971, 1972 and 1973) and should be consulted for further information and for references to original reports.

Drugs affected	*Drugs which interfere*	*Result of interaction*
ALIMENTARY SYSTEM		
Carbenoxolone	Spironolactone	Apparent inhibition of ulcer healing.
DRUGS ACTING ON THE HEART		
Digoxin **Digitoxin**	Diuretics: thiazides frusemide ethacrynic acid Carbenoxolone Amphotericin B	Toxicity increased by hypokalaemia.
	Suxamethonium	Increased risk of arrhythmias.
	Cholestyramine	Reduced absorption of digitoxin (and ? digoxin).
	Phenobarbitone Phenytoin Phenylbutazone	Reduced effect of digitoxin due to increased metabolism.

Drugs affected	*Drugs which interfere*	*Result of interaction*
Lignocaine	Phenytoin	Sino-atrial arrest.

ANTIHYPERTENSIVE DRUGS

Drugs affected	*Drugs which interfere*	*Result of interaction*
All	Phenylbutazone Corticosteroids Carbenoxolone Oral contraceptives	Hypotensive effect antagonised by drugs causing fluid retention or hypertension.
	Alcohol Sedatives and hypnotics Tranquillisers Antidepressants (but see below) L-dopa Fenfluramine Anaesthetics	Potentiation. These drugs all produce hypotension as a side effect.
Guanethidine **Bethanidine** **Debrisoquine**	Tricyclic antidepressants Indirect sympathomimetic amines Chlorpromazine?	Antagonism. Neuronal uptake to site of action prevented. N.B. Many proprietary common cold remedies contain indirect sympathomimetic amines, e.g. phenylpropanolamine, ephedrine.
Clonidine	Tricyclic antidepressants	Antagonism. Probably a central effect.
Methyldopa	Tricyclic antidepressants Phenothiazines	Hypertension may occur — possibly because uptake of α-methylnoradrenaline is prevented.

Drugs affected	*Drugs which interfere*	*Result of interaction*
DIURETICS		
Thiazides **Frusemide** **Ethacrynic acid**	Corticosteroids Carbenoxolone Phenylbutazone	Increased urinary potassium loss. Diuretic effect antagonised by fluid retention.
Spironolactone	Aspirin	Inhibition of natriuretic effect — mechanism unknown.
ORAL ANTICOAGULANTS		
Coumarins Warfarin	Cholestyramine	Reduced effect due to decreased absorption.
Dicoumarol Nicoumalone	Barbiturates Dichloralphenazone Glutethimide Methaqualone Phenytoin Carbamazepine Griseofulvin Rifampicin	Reduced effect due to increased metabolism. Overdose and bleeding may occur when the interacting drug is stopped.
	Vitamin K	Reversal of anticoagulant effect due to competitive inhibition. N.B. Some proprietary preparations for chilblains contain sufficient Vitamin K to inhibit the effect of oral anticoagulants (e.g. Adaprin, Amisyn, Pernivit).
	Phenylbutazone Oxyphenbutazone Mefenamic acid Chloral hydrate, triclofos	Increased effect due to displacement from protein binding. Phenylbutazone also inhibits metabolism.

Drugs affected	*Drugs which interfere*	*Result of interaction*
	Clofibrate	Increased effect — mechanism unclear but may be partly due to displacement from protein binding.
	Chloramphenicol Disulfiram Alcohol (acute intoxication) ? Allopurinol	Increased effect due to inhibition of metabolism.
	Anabolic steroids Oxymetholone Norethandrolone	Increased effect — possibly due to decreased receptor affinity for Vitamin K.
	Neomycin	Increased effect due to impaired absorption of Vitamin K — probably secondary to steatorrhoea.
	Salicylates ? p-Aminosalicylic acid Quinidine	Additive hypoprothrombinaemic effect. Aspirin also affects other aspects of haemostasis.
Phenindione (The indandione anticoagulants do not appear to share most of the coumarin inter-actions)	Clofibrate	Increased effect — mechanism unknown.
	Salicylates Neomycin	An increased effect should be anticipated.
	Vitamin K	Reversal of anticoagulant effect due to competitive inhibition (see under Coumarins above).

Drugs affected	*Drugs which interfere*	*Result of interaction*
ANALGESICS		
Aspirin	Alcohol	Increased risk of gastrointestinal bleeding.
Indomethacin	Aspirin	Impaired absorption and decreased effect have been reported but evidence is conflicting.
	Probenecid	Reduced renal excretion and increased clinical effect.
HYPNOTICS AND SEDATIVES		
Barbiturates **Other hypnotics** **Benzodiazepines**	Alcohol Narcotic analgesics Antihistamines Tranquillisers Antidepressants	Increased C.N.S. depression.
TRANQUILLISERS		
Chlorpromazine	Aluminium hydroxide Magnesium trisilicate Benzhexol	Absorption of chlorpromazine significantly reduced but clinical importance unknown.
ANTIDEPRESSANTS		
Tricyclic antidepressants	Barbiturates	Metabolism stimulated and plasma levels reduced, but clinical importance unknown.

Drugs affected	*Drugs which interfere*	*Result of interaction*
Monoamine oxidase inhibitors	Foods containing tyramine or dopamine, e.g. cheese, bovril.	Hypertensive crisis — severe headache — risk of subarachnoid haemorrhage.
N.B. Interactions may occur up to two weeks after stopping treatment with an MAOI	Indirect sympathomimetic amines: amphetamine ephedrine phenylpropanolamine phenylephrine metaraminol L-dopa	
	Tricyclic antidepressants	CNS excitation, hypertension and convulsions.
	Pethidine	CNS excitation, hypertension or hypotension, coma.
	Reserpine	CNS excitation and hypertension.
LITHIUM CARBONATE		
	Sodium bicarbonate Acetazolamide Aminophylline	Increased excretion of lithium. Clinical significance unknown.
	Diuretics	Lithium excretion is reduced in patients on thiazide diuretics. Lithium toxicity is increased by sodium depletion.
ANTICONVULSANTS		
All	Phenothiazines Tricyclic antidepressants	Reduced effect — due to lowering of con vulsive threshold.

Drugs affected	*Drugs which interfere*	*Result of interaction*
Phenytoin	Isoniazid Sulthiame Disulfiram Dicoumarol Chloramphenicol	Potentiation and increased toxicity due to inhibition of metabolism.
	Phenobarbitone Carbamazepine	Metabolism stimulated but clinical significance small.
ANTI-PARKINSON DRUGS		
Anticholinergic drugs Benzhexol Orphenadrine Benztropine, etc.	Tricyclic antidepressants Phenothiazines Antihistamines Monamine oxidase inhibitors	Increased anticholinergic side effects — dry mouth, blurred vision, urinary retention, etc.
	Tricyclic antidepressants ? Monoamine oxidase inhibitors	Excitement and confusion.
L-dopa	Phenothiazines Reserpine Methyldopa Butyrophenones Metoclopramide	Antagonised. These drugs have extrapyramidal side effects.
	Pyridoxine (present in many proprietary multi-vitamin preparations)	Antagonised — reversal of therapeutic effect.
MUSCLE RELAXANTS		
All	Antibiotics— aminoglycosides colistin Quinidine Phenytoin Propranolol (large doses)	Increased or prolonged paralysis. These drugs have neuromuscular blocking activity.

Drugs affected	*Drugs which interfere*	*Result of interaction*
Competitive neuromuscular blockers—		
Tubocurarine Gallamine Pancuronium	Ether	Increased neuromuscular blockade — additive effect.
	Diuretics Carbenoxolone	Potentiation by hypokalaemia is a probable, but poorly documented risk.
Depolarising neuromuscular blockers—		
Suxamethonium	Neostigmine Ecothiopate eye-drops Cyclophosphamide Thiotepa ? Phenelzine	Potentiation — prolonged paralysis. These drugs have anticholinesterase activity.
	Propanidid	Potentiation — mechanism not established.
	Digoxin	Increased risk of arrhythmias.
ANAESTHETICS		
All	Antihypertensive drugs	Potentiation of hypotensive effect.
	β-adrenergic blockers e.g. propranolol practolol	Potentiation of hypotensive effect. Loss of compensatory reflex tachycardia.
	Chlorpromazine	Potentiation of hypotensive effect. Vasopressors ineffective because chlorpromazine block α-adrenergic receptors.
Ether	Tubocurarine Antibiotics — aminoglycosides colistin	Increased nueromuscular blockade — additive effect.

Drugs affected	*Drugs which interfere*	*Result of interaction*
Halothane **Cyclopropane** **Trichlorethylene** **(Methoxyflurane)**	Adrenaline Isoprenaline	Cardiac arrythmias may occur due to increased sensitivity of the myocardium to catecholamines.
Methoxyflurane	Tetracyclines	Increased risk of polyuric renal failure.
VASOCONSTRICTORS		
Noradrenaline **Adrenaline**	Tricyclic antidepressants	Potentiation due to inhibition of neuronal uptake. Hypertension, tachycardia, arrhythmias may occur.
	Guanethidine Reserpine	Potentiation due to increased receptor sensitivity ("denervation supersensitivity").
Metaraminol **Phenylephrine**	Guanethidine Reserpine Debrisoquine	Potentiation of direct vasoconstrictor effect. Hypertension may occur. N.B. Phenylephrine is present in many proprietary common cold remedies.
ANTIBACTERIAL DRUGS		
Phenoxymethylpenicillin	Neomycin	Reduced absorption.
Tetracyclines	Oral iron preparations, Calcium, magnesium and aluminium salts (e.g. antacids)	Absorption reduced due to chelation.
Lincomycin	Kaolin mixtures	Reduced absorption.

Drugs affected	*Drugs which interfere*	*Result of interaction*
Streptomycin **Neomycin** **Kanamycin** **Gentamicin**	Frusemide Ethacrynic acid	Increased risk of ototoxicity.
Cephaloridine	Frusemide Ethacrynic acid	Increased risk of nephrotoxicity.
Nitrofurantoin	Probenecid	Renal excretion is decreased — increased toxicity is a possibility.
Rifampicin	p-Aminosalicylic acid	Reduced absorption.
p-Aminosalicylic acid	Probenecid	Decreased renal excretion — increased toxicity.
Isoniazid	p-Aminosalicylic	Acetylation inhibited— blood levels increased.
OTHER ANTIMICROBIAL DRUGS		
Griseofulvin	Phenobarbitone	Reduced effect due to increased metabolism and/or reduced absorption.
Metronidazole	Alcohol	"Antabuse-like" reaction due to inhibition of aldehyde dehydrogenase.
Dapsone	Probenecid	Renal excretion decreased — increased risk of haemolytic anaemia.
HORMONES		
Corticosteroids (all)	Diuretics Thiazides Frusemide Ethacrynic acid	Increased potassium loss and hypokalaemia.

Drugs affected	*Drugs which interfere*	*Result of interaction*
	Phenobarbitone Phenytoin Rifampicin	Increased metabolism of hydrocortisone and ? prednisone, with loss of therapeutic effect.
Dexamethasone	Phenobarbitone Phenytoin	Increased metabolism of dexamethasone and failure to suppress pituitary during dexamethasone suppression test.
Thyroxine	Cholestyramine	Absorption reduced.
	Phenytoin	Thyroxine displaced from protein-binding. False low PBI. Possible transient increase in effect.
DRUGS USED IN DIABETES		
All	Alcohol MAOIs Propranolol Aspirin (large doses)	Hypoglycaemia potentiated and prolonged
	Corticosteroids Thiazide diuretics ? Phenytoin ? Isoniazid	These drugs produce hyperglycaemia and antagonise anti-diabetic drugs.
Sulphonylureas Chlorpropamide Tolbutamide	Chloramphenicol Dicoumarol Phenylbutazone Sulphaphenazole	Potentiation of hypoglycaemia; mainly due to inhibition of metabolism. Renal excretion may be inhibited by phenylbutazone. Phenylbutazone and sulphaphenazole displace tolbutamide from protein-binding.

continued next page

Drugs affected	*Drugs which interfere*	*Result of interaction*
	Alcohol	"Antabuse effect" — flushing, sweating, tachycardia.
Biguanides Phenformin (Metformin)	Alcohol	Increased risk of lactic acidosis.
CYTOTOXIC DRUGS		
Mercaptopurine **Azathioprine**	Allopurinol	Potentiation and increased toxicity due to inhibition of metabolism by xanthine oxidase.
Methotrexate	Salicylates	Decreased renal excretion and displacement from protein binding may increase toxicity. Clinical importance unknown.
Procarbazine	Alcohol	"Antabuse-like" reaction due to inhibition of aldehyde dehydrogenase.
ORAL IRON PREPARATIONS		
All	Magnesium trisilicate (? other antacids) Tetracyclines	Reduced absorption.
DRUGS USED IN GOUT		
Probenecid **Sulfinpyrazone**	Aspirin (less than 2g daily)	Uricosuric effect inhibited.

continued next page

Drugs affected	*Drugs which interfere*	*Result of Interaction*
ALCOHOL		
(Most of these interactions appear elsewhere in the appendix but are summarised here for convenience)	Disulfiram Metronidazole Furazolidine Procarbazine	"Antabuse" reaction due to inhibition of aldehyde dehydrogenase.
	Sulphonylureas (especially chlorpropamide)	Reaction similar to "Antabuse" reaction — probably not due to inhibition of aldehyde dehydrogenase.
	Tolbutamide Phenytoin Warfarin Pentobarbitone	Prolonged heavy alcohol intake produces enzyme induction and increased metabolism. Acute alcohol intoxication may inhibit the metabolism of the same drugs.
	Hypnotics, sedatives, tranquillisers, antidepressants, narcotic analgesics, antihistamines	Sedative effect is potentiated by alcohol.
	MAOIs	Some alcoholic drinks contain enough tyramine to produce a hypertensive crisis.
	Antihypertensive drugs	Increased hypotension due to vasodilator effect of alcohol.
	Phenformin ? Metformin	Increased risk of lactic acidosis.

APPENDIX IV

DRUGS IN PREGNANCY

CARDIOVASCULAR SYSTEM

ANTIHYPERTENSIVE DRUGS

Reserpine	Given within a few days before delivery may cause neonatal bradycardia, nasal stuffiness, and drowsiness.
Diazoxide	Prolonged use may produce diabetes in the fetus. Emergency use in toxaemia appears to be safe, but inhibition of uterine activity may produce temporary cessation of labour.

DIURETICS

Thiazides	May produce neonatal thrombocytopenic purpura if given during the last three months of pregnancy.

ANTICOAGULANTS

Coumarins Warfarin Dicoumarol **Phenindione**	Foetal or neonatal haemorrhage and death may occur. Heparin should be substituted during the last three weeks of pregnancy.

NERVOUS SYSTEM

ANALGESICS

Aspirin	In two recent surveys (Nelson and Forfar, 1971; Richards, 1969) mothers of infants with congenital malformations were more

likely to have taken aspirin in early pregnancy than a control group of mothers with normal infants. However, a causal relationship has not been established and the risk is likely to be small. Given in late pregnancy large doses of aspirin may produce hypoprothrombinaemia and foetal or neonatal haemorrhage. It displaces bilirubin from protein-binding and may produce kernicterus in the neonate.

Phenacetin	May produce haemolysis or methaemoglobinaemia in the neonate if given in late pregnancy.
Amidopyrine	Fatal agranulocytosis has occurred in the newborn as a result of administration of amidopyrine to the mother before delivery.
Indomethacin	Displaces bilirubin from protein-binding and may produce kernicterus in the neonate if given in late pregnancy.
Narcotic analgesics Heroin Pethidine Morphine Methadone	Given during labour these may cause respiratory depression in the newborn. Babies born to mothers dependent on narcotics may be premature and may show a physical withdrawal syndrome with hyperirritability, high pitched cry, respiratory distress, vomiting, diarrhoea and dehydration. Perinatal mortality is increased.

HYPNOTICS AND SEDATIVES

All may depress fetal respiration if given to the mother during labour.

Barbiturates	A neonatal withdrawal syndrome may occur in babies born to mothers taking a barbiturate during the last trimester of pregnancy.
Diazepam	Neonatal hypotonia and hypothermia if large amounts given during labour. (More than 30 mg)
Thalidomide	High incidence of severe congenital malformations if taken during first three months.

TRICYCLIC ANTIDEPRESSANTS

Imipramine **Amitriptyline** **Nortriptyline**	Congenital malformations have been reported but a causal relationship has not been established. Withdrawal symptoms have been described in infants whose mothers received imipramine or desmethylimipramine during pregnancy.

LITHIUM CARBONATE

Congenital malformations have been reported and lithium is best avoided during the first three months. Renal lithium clearance increases during pregnancy and falls at delivery. Close monitoring of maternal blood levels is necessary to maintain therapeutic levels and avoid neonatal toxicity.

ANTICONVULSANTS

Phenobarbitone **Phenytoin** **Primidone** **Trimethadione**	The incidence of congenital malformations appears to be increased. This may be associated with folic acid deficiency and adequate folate supplements should be given during pregnancy. A coagulation defect sometimes occurs resulting in neonatal haemorrhage.

STIMULANTS

Dexamphetamine	An increased incidence of congenital malformations — particularly congenital heart disease — has been reported.
Lysergic acid diethylamide LSD	May be associated with increased incidence of spontaneous abortion. Chromosome abnormalities may occur but evidence that it produces congenital malformations is conflicting.

MUSCLE RELAXANTS AND THEIR ANTAGONISTS

Tubocurarine	Large doses given during labour may produce paralysis at birth, but usual doses appear to be harmless.
Neostigmine **Pyridostigmine**	Large doses may produce a neonatal myasthenic syndrome.

ANAESTHETICS

Gaseous anaesthetics **Thiopentone**	May produce respiratory depression in the neonate if used during labour.

LOCAL ANAESTHETICS

Procaine **Prilocaine**	May produce methaemoglobinaemia in the neonate if used during labour.
Bupivicaine	May produce fetal bradycardia following paracervical block anaesthesia.

GENITAL SYSTEM

SEX HORMONES

Androgens	May produce virilisation of female fetus if given during first three months of pregnancy.
Progestogens	
Ethisterone Norethisterone Hydroxyprogesterone caproate Dydrogesterone Norethynodrel	May produce virilisation of female fetus when used to prevent abortion in early pregnancy. The small doses present in oral contraceptives are unlikely to have this effect.
Oestrogens Stilboestrol	Use in early pregnancy has been associated with virilisation of female fetus. Recent reports suggest an increased incidence of carcinoma of the vagina in girls aged 16-20 whose mothers took stilboestrol during pregnancy.
Progestogen/Oestrogen combinations	
Oral contraceptives	An increased incidence of congenital malformations has been reported in offspring of women who took these in early pregnancy, but the evidence is inconclusive.

Pregnancy test, e.g. Primidos, Amenorone	A possible association with meningomyelocele has been reported, and preliminary results of a case-control study by the Committee on Safety of Medicines suggest that the use of these preparations could occasionally lead to abnormalities in the fetus.
Gonadotrophins	
Chorionic Gonadotrophin, Human FSH, Clomiphene	Multiple pregnancies may occur when these are used to induce ovulation in the treatment of infertility. A possible association with anencephaly has been reported.

INFECTIONS

ANTIBACTERIAL DRUGS

Tetracyclines (all)	Chelate with calcium and are deposited in developing bones and teeth. Transient inhibition of bone growth may occur. Discoloration of the deciduous teeth occurs from the 14th week of pregnancy and the permanent teeth are affected during the last three months. Enamel hypoplasia may increase susceptibility to dental caries.
Chloramphenicol	If given just before term, may produce circulatory collapse (grey syndrome) in the neonate due to immaturity of hepatic conjugating enzymes.
Aminoglycosides	
Streptomycin, Dihydrostreptomycin, Gentamicin, Kanamycin	May cause auditory or vestibular nerve damage. Serious damage appears to be rare.

Sulphonamides	May produce kernicterus, haemolysis or methaemoglobinaemia in the neonate if given in late pregnancy.
Co-trimoxazole	May interfere with folate metabolism and is best avoided in pregnancy (see also sulphonamides).
Nitrofurantoin	May produce haemolysis in the neonate if given in late pregnancy.
Novobiocin	May produce kernicterus in the neonate if given in late pregnancy.

ANTITUBERCULOUS DRUGS

Ethionamide	One small survey (Potworowska, 1966) showed an increased incidence of congenital malformations, but this has not been confirmed.

ANTIMALARIAL DRUGS

Chloroquine	May cause congenital deafness. Concentrated in fetal eye; theoretical risk of retinal damage.
Quinine	Large doses in early pregnancy may produce abortion. Congenital deafness and hypoplasia of the optic nerve have been reported.
Pyrimethamine	Interferes with folate metabolism and is best avoided in pregnancy.
Primaquine	May produce haemolysis in the neonate if given in late pregnancy.

METABOLISM

CORTICOSTEROIDS

Cortisone **Prednisone** **Prednisolone** **Dexamethazone**	Cortisone is teratogenic in animals. It is possible that large doses of corticosteroids given in early pregnancy may very rarely produce congenital malformations in man. An increased incidence of stillbirth and fetal distress has been reported in association with prednisolone given during pregnancy.

DRUGS USED IN THYROID DISEASE

Radioactive iodine	May damage fetal thyroid and cause hypothyroidism if given after the first three months.
Methylthiouracil **Thiouracil** **Carbimazole**	May produce goitre in the foetus. Neonatal hypothyroidism may occur but is usually mild and transient. It is best to withdraw these drugs four weeks before delivery.
Iodides (present in many cough mixtures)	May produce goitre and neonatal hypothyroidism. Although the goitre disappears spontaneously mental retardation may occur if replacement therapy is not given.
Sulphonylureas	
Chlorpropamide Tolbutamide Glibenclamide	The incidence of congenital malformations does not appear to be increased in infants born to mothers who have taken these throughout pregnancy. Neonatal hypoglycaemia may occur,

and oral therapy should be stopped at least three days before delivery. Tolbutamide displaces bilirubin from protein-binding and may produce kernicterus in the neonate.

MALIGNANT DISEASE AND IMMUNOSUPPRESSANTS

Folic acid antagonists Methotrexate Aminopterin **Cyclophosphamide** **Busulphan** **Chlorambucil** **Melphalan** **Vincristine, vinblastine** **Daunorubicin**	High incidence of spontaneous abortion and fetal malformations. The folic acid antagonists are the most likely to damage the fetus.
Azathioprine **Mercaptopurine**	Also produce spontaneous abortion and fetal malformations but the risk appears to be less than with other cytotoxic drugs. There are many reports of normal babies born to mothers taking azathioprine during pregnancy.

VITAMINS

Vitamin A	Large doses are teratogenic in animals. There is some evidence that this may also be true in man.
Vitamin D	It is possible that idiopathic hypercalcaemia of infancy may sometimes be associated with a high intake of Vitamin D during pregnancy, but this is unproven.

Vitamin K

Menaphthone Acetomenaphthone Menadiol sodium phosphate	Excessive doses given before delivery to prevent haemorrhagic disease of the newborn may produce haemolysis. Menadiol sodium phosphate displaces bilirubin from protein-binding and kernicterus may occur.

VACCINES

Rubella Vaccine	Vaccination frequently produces a viraemia and virus has been recovered from the placenta and foetal tissues after vaccination. The risk of congenital malformations occurring is unknown, but vaccination should not be carried out during pregnancy.
Smallpox Vaccine	Primary vaccination may produce a viraemia and fetal vaccinia may result in abortion or stillbirth. Vaccination during pregnancy should only be carried out if absolutely necessary.

LACTATION

Drugs excreted in the milk which may harm the child include:

Iodides **Radioactive iodine** **Thiouracils**	May produce hypothyroidism and neonatal goitre.
Bromides	Rashes and drowsiness.
Oral anticoagulants	Haemorrhage has been reported.
Phenobarbitone **Phenytoin**	Drowsiness.

Diazepam	Pharmacological amounts appear in breast-milk and may produce drowsiness.
Lithium	Probably harmless if maternal blood levels well-controlled.
Ergotamine	Ergotism may occur.
Diazoxide	Appears in breast-milk but risk to infants unknown.
Alcohol	Large amounts may affect the infant.
Penicillin	Small amounts are excreted in breast-milk and may be sufficient to produce hypersensitivity.
Tetracycline **Chloramphenicol**	Excreted in breast-milk in sufficient amounts to produce a pharmacological effect.

REFERENCES

Alexanderson, B., Evans, D. A. P. and Sjöqvist, F. (1969). Steady state plasma levels of nortriptyline in twins: influence of genetic factors and drug therapy. Brit. med. J., **4**, 764.

Almeyda, J. and Baker, H. (1970). Adverse reactions to hypoglycaemic agents. Brit. J. Dermatol., **82**, 634.

Almeyda, J. and Baker, H. (1971). Cutaneous reactions to anti-rheumatic drugs. Brit. J. Dermatol., **84**, 707.

Almeyda, J. and Baker, H. (1971). Cutaneous reactions to imipramine and chlordiazepoxide. Brit. J. Dermatol., **84**, 298.

Almeyda, J. and Levantine, A. (1972). Cutaneous reactions to barbiturates, chloral hydrate and its derivatives. Brit. J. Dermatol., **86**, 313.

Almeyda, J. and Levantine, A. (1973). Cutaneous reactions to cardiovascular drugs. Brit. J. Dermatol., **88**, 313.

Almeyda, J. and Levantine, A. (1971). Lichenoid drug eruptions. Brit. J. Dermatol., **85**, 604.

American Pharmaceutical Association. (1973). Evaluations of Drug interactions.

Annotation. (1889). Hyderabad Medical School. Chloroform inhalation. Lancet, **i**, 394.

Ashton, H. (1971). Drugs and the foetus and neonate. Adverse Drug Reaction Bulletin, **28**, 80.

Bahn, S. L. (1972). Drug related dental destruction. Oral surg., Oral med., Oral pathol., **33**, 49.

Baker, H. and Levene, G. M. (1969). Cutaneous reactions to anti-coagulants. Brit. J. Dermatol., **81**, 236.

Baker, H. and Moore-Robinson, M. (1970). Cutaneous responses to aspirin and its derivatives. Brit. J. Dermatol., **82**, 319.

Balasubramaniam, K., Mawer, G. E., Pohl, J. E. F. and Simons, P. J. G. (1972). Impairment of cognitive function association with hydroxyamylobarbitone accumulation in patients with renal insufficiency. Br. J. Pharmacol., **45**, 360.

Beeley, L., Bishop, J. M., Leach, R. H. and Walker, G. F. (1974). A real time system for drug prescribing. Symposium on medical data processing. Toulouse, March 1974.

Boakes, A. J., Laurence, D. R., Lovel, K. W., O'Neill, R. and Verrill, P. J. (1972). Adverse reactions to local anaesthetic/vasoconstrictor preparations. Brit. Dent. J., **133**, 137.

Boakes, A. J., Laurence, D. R., Teoh, P. C., Barar, F. S. K., Benedikter, L. T. and Prichard, B. N. C. (1973). Interactions between sympathomimetic amines and antidepressant agents in man. Brit. med. J., **1**, 311.

Boman, G., Hanngren, A., Malmborg, A. S., Bőrga, O. and Sjöqvist, F. (1971). Drug interaction: decreased serum concentration of Rifampicin when given with P.A.S. Lancet, **i**, 800.

Boston Collaborative Drug Surveillance Program. (1972). Relation between digoxin arrhythmias and ABO blood groups. Circulation, **45**, 352.

Breckenridge, A. and Orme, M. L. E. (1973). Measurement of plasma warfarin concentrations in clinical practice in: Biological effects of drugs in relation to their plasma concentration. Ed. Davies, D. S. and Prichard, B. N. C., Macmillan.

Bruinsma, W. (1973). A guide to drug eruptions. Excerpta Medica.

Clarke, C. A., Evans, D. A. P., Harris, R., McConnell, R. B. and Woodrow, J. C. (1968). Genetics in medicine: a review, Part II. Pharmacogenetics. Quart. J. Med., **37**, 183.

Colebrook, L. and Kenny, M. (1936). Treatment of human puerperal infections and of experimental infections in mice with Prontosil. Lancet, **i**, 1279.

Connell, P. H. (1958). Amphetamine psychoses. Maudlsey Monograph, No. 5. London, Chapman and Hall.

Crooks, J., Clark, C. G., Caie, H. B. and Mawson, W. B. (1965). Prescribing and Administration of Drugs in Hospital. Lancet, **i**, 373.

Crooks, J., Weir, R. D., Coull, D. C., McNab, J. W., Calder, G., Barnett, J. W. and Caie, H. B. (1967). Evaluation of a method of prescribing drugs in hospital, and a new method of recording their administration. Lancet, **i**, 668.

de Stevens, G. (1971). In: Decision-making on the efficacy and safety of drugs. Ed. Cooper, J. D. Interdisciplinary Communication Associates Inc. Washington, D.C., U.S.A.

Daniels, M. and Hill, A. B. (1952). Chemotherapy of pulmonary tuberculosis in young adults; an analysis of the combined results of three Medical Research Council trials. Brit. med. J., **1**, 1162.

Dodds, E. C., Golberg, L., Lawson, W., and Robinson, R. (1938). Oestrogenic activity of alkylated stilboestrols. Nature, **142**, 34.

Dower, F. H. and Stevenson, C. J. (1973). Contact dermatitis from topical drugs. Adverse drug reaction bulletin, **42**, 136.

Editorial. (1969). Drugs and the eye—Parts I & II. Adverse drug reaction bulletin. Nos. 17 and 18.

Engels, A. and Siderius, P. (1968). The consumption of drugs. Report of a study, 1966–7. Unpublished. W.H.O. working document. EURO. 3101, Copenhagen.

Evered, D. and Hall, R. (1972). Drugs and the endocrine system. Adverse drug reaction bulletin, **34**, 104.

Feinmann, L. (1974). Drug-induced lung disease. Adverse drug reaction bulletin, **45**, 148.

Gibson, J. S. and Wade, O. L. (1964). Dealing with drug dependence. Prescribers Journal, **4**, 88.

Gilgore, S. G. (1971). In: Decision-making on the efficacy and safety of drugs. Ed. Cooper, J. D. Interdisciplinary Communication Associates Inc. Washington, D.C., U.S.A.

Girdwood, R. H. (Ed.). (1973). Blood disorders due to drugs and other agents. Excerpta Medica.

Hansten, P. D. (1973). Drug interactions. Lea and Febiger.

Hoddinott, B. C., Gowdey, C. W., Coulter, W. K. and Parker, J. M. (1967). Drug reactions and errors in administration on a medical ward. Canad. med. Ass. J., **97**, 1001.

Hood, H. and Wade, O. L. (1968). Use of amphetamines in general practice. Lancet, **ii**, 96.

Hurwitz, N. (1969). Predisposing factors in adverse reactions to drugs. Brit. med. J., **1**, 536.

Hurwitz , N. and Wade, O. L. (1969). Intensive hospital monitoring of adverse reactions to drugs. Brit. med. J., **1**, 531.

Huxley, A. (1937). Ends and Means. Chatto and Windus, 1937.

Inman, W. H. W. and Vessey, M. P. (1968). Investigation of deaths from pulmonary, coronary and cerebral thrombosis and embolism in women of child bearing age. Brit. med. J., **2**, 193.

Kerr, D. N. S. and Walls, J. (1970). Renal damage due to drugs. Adverse drug reaction bulletin, **20** and **21**, 54.

Knowles, John A. (1965). Excretion of drugs in milk—a review. J. Paediatrics, **66**, 1068.

Krache, R. R. and Parker, F. P. (1934). The etiology of granulopaenia (agranulocytosis). J. Lab. Clin. Med., **19**, 799.

Kutt, H., Brennen, R., Dehejia, H. and Verebely, K. (1970). Diphenylhydantoin intoxication. A complication of Isoniazid therapy. Amer. Rev. Resp. Dis., **101**, 377.

Lawrie, E., Brunton, J. L., Bomford, G. and Hakim, R. D. (1890). Report of the Second Hyderabad Chloroform Commission. Lancet, **i**, 149.

Leader, (1889). The Hyderabad Commission on Chloroform. Lancet, **i**, 438.

Leading Article. (1973). Drug induced respiratory disorders. Brit. med. J., **2**, 320.

Leading Article. (1973). Safe prescribing in liver disease. Brit. med. J., **2**, 193.

Levantine, A. and Almeyda, J. (1972). Cutaneous reactions to anticonvulsants. Brit. J. Dermatol., **87**, 646.

Levantine, A. and Almeyda, J. (1972). Cutaneous reactions to antituberculous drugs. Brit. J. Dermatol., **86**, 651.

Levantine, A. and Almeyda, J. (1973). Drug-induced alopecia. Brit. J. Dermatol., **89**, 549.

Levantine, A. and Almeyda, J. (1973). Drug-induced changes in pigmentation. Brit. J. Dermatol., **89,** 105.

Lewis, P., Jick, H., Slone, D. and Shapiro, S. (1971). The role of genetic factors and serum protein binding in determining drug response as revealed by comprehensive drug surveillance. Ann. N.Y. Acad Sci., **179,** 729.

Louis, P. C. A. (1828). Memoires et observations. Recherches sur les effects de la saignée dans plusiers maladies inflammatoires. Archiv. Gen. Med., **18,** 322.

Louis, P. C. A. (1835). Recherches sur les effects de la saignée. Paris, Bailliere.

Lowe, C. R. (1973). Congenital malformations among infants born to epileptic women. Lancet, **i, 9.**

McClelland, H. A. (1973). Psychiatric complications of drug therapy. Adverse Drug Reaction Bulletin, **40,** 128.

McDonald, S. (1918). Acute yellow atrophy in syphilis. Brit. med. J., **1,** 76.

McKendrick, J. G., Coats, J. and Newman, D. (1880). Report on the action of anaesthetics. Brit. med. J., **2,** 957.

Madison, F. W. and Squier, T. L. (1933). Primary granulocytopaenia after administration of drugs containing a benzene chain. Annual meeting of Central Society for Medical Research, Chicago, Oct. 1933. Quoted by Krache, R. R. and Parker, F. P. (1934). Loc. cit.

Manninen, V., Apajalahti, A., Melin, J. and Karesoja, M. (1973). Altered absorption of digoxin in patients given propantheline and metoclopramide. Lancet, **i,** 398.

Maxwell, J. D. and Williams, R. (1971). Adverse drug reactions and the liver. Adverse drug reaction bulletin, **29,** 84.

Medical Research Council. (1963). Assessment of drug toxicity. International paper 63/658.

Medical Research Council. (1922). Toxic effect following employment of arsenobenzenol preparations. Special report series, No. 66.

Mellin, G. W. and Katzenstein, M. (1962). Saga of thalidomide. New Eng. J. Med., **267,** 1184.

Meyler, L. and Herxheimer, A. (Ed). (1968). Side effects of drugs, Vol. 6. Excerpta Medica.

Meyler, L. and Herxheimer, A. (Ed.). (1972). Side effects of drugs, Vol. 7. Excerpta Medica.

Meyler, L. and Peck, H. M. (Ed.). (1972). Drug-induced diseases, Vol. 4. Excerpta Medica.

Misage, R. and McDonald, R. H. (1970). Antagonism of hypotensive action of bethanidine by "common cold remedy". Brit. med. J. **4,** 347.

Moorhead, N. C. (1968). Amphetamine consumption in Northern Ireland. J. Irish. Med. Ass., **61,** 80.

Mushin, A. S. (1972). Ocular damage by drugs in children. Adverse drug reaction bulletin, **36,** 112.

Nelson, M. M. and Forfar, J. O. (1971). Associations between drugs administered during pregnancy and congenital abnormalities of the fetus. Brit. med. J., **1**, 523.

Neuvonen, P. J., Gothoni, G., Hackman, R. and af Bjorksten, K. (1970). Interference of iron with the absorption of tetracyclines in man. Brit. med. J., **4**, 532.

Nimmo, J., Heading, R. C., Tothill, P. and Prescott, L. F. (1973). Pharmacological modification of gastric emptying: effects of propantheline and metoclopramide on paracetoamol absorption. Brit. med. J., **1**, 587.

O'Malley, K., Crooks, J., Duke, E. and Stevenson, I. H. (1971). Effect of age and sex on human drug metabolism. Brit. med. J., **3**, 607.

O'Reilly, R. A. and Aggeler, P. M. (1970). Determinants of the response to oral anticoagulants in man. Pharmacological Reviews, **22**, 35.

Oates, J. A., Mitchell, J. R., Feagin, O. T., Kaufmann, J. S. and Shand, D. G. (1971). Distribution of Guanidium antihypertensives; mechanism of their selective action. Annals of N.Y. Academy of Sciences, **179**, 302.

Pool, J. G., O'Reilly, R. A., Schneiderman, L. J. and Alexander, M. (1968). Warfarin resistance in the rat. Amer. J. Physiol., **215**, 627.

Rake, G. W. (1927). A case of subacute yellow atrophy following the taking of atophan. Guy's Hosp. Rep. **77**, 229.

Report of Royal Commission. (1874). On the practice of subjecting live animals to experiments for scientific purposes.

Richards, I. D. G. (1969). Congenital malformations and environmental influences in pregnancy. Brit. J. Prev. Soc. Med., **23**, 218.

Rogers, S. C. (1967). Imipramine and benzhexol. Brit. med. J., **1**, 500.

Royal College of Physicians. (1973). Report of Committee on the supervision of the ethics of clinical research investigations in institutions. London.

Seidl, L. G., Thornton, G. F., Smith, J. W. and Cluff, L. E. (1966). Studies of the epidemiology of adverse drug reactions III. Reactions in patients on a general medical service. Bull., Johns Hopk. Hosp., **119**, 299.

Short, C. L. and Baker, W. (1933). Cinocophen hypersensitiveness. Ann. int. Med., **6**, 1449.

Sjöqvist, F., Alexanderson, B., Åsberg, M., Bertilsson, L., Borgå, O., Hamberger, B. and Tuck, D. (1971). Pharmacokinetics and biological effects of nortriptyline in man. Acta. Pharmacologica et Toxicologica, 29, Suppl. 3, 255.

Smith, R. N. (1972). Generic equivalence and non-equivalence of drugs. Lancet, **ii**, 528.

South, J. (1972). Teratogenic effect of anticonvulsants. Lancet, **ii**, 1154.

Speidel, B. D. and Meadow, S. R. (1972). Maternal epilepsy and abnormalities of the fetus and newborn. Lancet, **ii**, 839.

Stockley, I. H. (1971). Interactions between the hypoglycaemic agents and other drugs. Pharm. J., **207,** 37.

Stockley, I. H. (1972). Drug-alcohol interactions. Pharm. J., **208,** 16.

Stockley, I. H. (1971). Interactions of digitalis and antiarrhythmic agents. Pharm. J., **207,** 179.

Stockley, I. H. (1973). Interactions of neuromuscular blockers, analgesics and anti-inflammatory agents. Pharm. J., **211,** 152.

Stockley, I. H. (1972). Interactions with antihypertensive agents. Pharm. J., **209,** 445.

Stockley, I. H. (1973). Interactions with anti-infective agents. Pharm. J., **210,** 36 and 62.

Stockley, I. H. (1973). Interactions with oral anticoagulants. Pharm. J., **210,** 339 and 395.

Stockley, I. H. (1972). Interactions with phenytoin, phenobarbitone and other anti-epileptic agents. Pharm. J., **209,** 105.

Stockley, I. H. (1973). Miscellaneous interactions: antineoplastics, cholestyramine, uricosuric agents and other drugs. Pharm. J., **211,** 175.

Stockley, I. H. (1973). Monoamine oxidase inhibitors: Part I—interactions with sympathomimetic agents. Pharm. J., **210,** 590.

Stockley, I. H. (1973). Monoamine oxidase inhibitors: Part II—interactions with antihypertensive agents, hypoglycaemics, CNS depressants, narcotics and antiparkinsoniam agents. Pharm. J., **211,** 95.

Stockley, I. H. (1972). Tricyclic antidepressants: Part I—Interactions with drugs affecting adrenergic neurones. Part II—General drug interactions. Pharm. J., **208,** 559 and 580.
Practolol produces psoriasiform rashes, conjunctival scarring, corneal opacities, positive LE cells and ANF, and fibrous peritonitis.

Thomsen, P. E. B., Ostenfeld, H. O. L. and Kristensen, M. (1970). Klorporpamid—fenylbutazon som arsag til hypoglykaemi. Ugeskr. Laeg., **132,** 1722.

Tyrer, J. H., Eadie, M. J., Sutherland, J. M. and Hooper, W. D. (1970). Outbreak of anticonvulsant intoxication in an Australian city. Brit. med. J., **4,** 271.

Vessell, E. S., Passananant i, G. T., Greene, F. E. and Page, J. G. (1971). Genetic control of drug levels and of the induction of drug metabolising enzymes in man. Ann. N.Y. Acad. Sci., **179,** 752.

Wade, O. L. (1972). Drug therapy in the elderly. Age and ageing. **1,** 65.

Wade, O. L. (1966). Prescribing of chloramphenicol and aplastic anaemia. J. Coll. gen. Practit., **12,** 277.

Wade, O. L., Hadden, D. R. and Hood, H. (1973). The prescribing of drugs used in the treatment of diabetes. Brit. J. prev. Soc. Med., **27,** 44.

Wade, O. L. and Hood, H. (1972). Prescribing of drugs reported to cause adverse reactions. Brit. J. Prev. Soc. Med., **26**, 205.

Wade, O. L. and Hood, H. (1972). Analysis of prescribing of an hypnotic in the community. Brit. J. Prev. Soc. Med., **26**, 2.

W.H.O. (1969). International drug monitoring. W.H.O. pilot research project. DMO/69.3. Geneva.

W.H.O. (1969). International drug monitoring. W.H.O. tech. Rep. Ser. No. 425. Geneva.

Wilson, J. G. (1973). Present status of drugs as teratogens in man. Teratology, **7**, 3–16.

Worster-Drought, C. (1923). Atophan poisoning. Brit. med. J., **1**, 148.

Yunis, A. A. (1973). In: Blood disorders due to drugs and other agents. Ed. Girdwood, R. H. Excertpa Medica, 107.

INDEX

For drugs see Drug Index pages 219–230

DRUG INDEX